ENDOCRINE
PROBLEMS

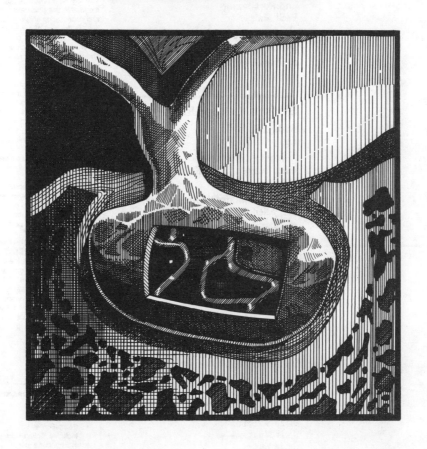

Nurse Review

Springhouse Corporation Book Division

Chairman
Eugene W. Jackson

Vice-Chairman
Daniel L. Cheney

President
Warren R. Erhardt

Vice-President and Director
William L. Gibson

Vice-President, Production and Purchasing
Bacil Guiley

Program Director
Jean Robinson

Art Director
John Hubbard

Staff for this section

Book Editor
Kathy Goldberg

Clinical Editor
Diane Schweisguth, RN, BSN, CCRN, CEN

Drug Information Manager
Larry Neil Gever, RPh, PharmD

Designer
Lynn Foulk Purvis

Illustrators
Julia DeVito
Dan Fione
Robert Jackson
Robert Neumann

Project Coordinator
Aline S. Miller

Production Coordinator
Maureen B. Carmichael

Editorial Services Manager
David R. Moreau

Copy Editors
Diane M. Labus
Doris Weinstock
Debra Young

Art Production Manager
Robert Perry

Artists
Mary Stangl

Typography Manager
David C. Kosten

Typography Assistants
Alicia Dempsey
Elizabeth A. DiCicco
Diane Paluba
Nancy Wirs

Senior Production Manager
Deborah C. Meiris

Assistant Production Managers
Pat Dorshaw
T.A. Landis

Clinical Consultants for this section

Joann M. Eland, RN, MA, PhD
Associate Professor of Nursing, University of Iowa, Iowa City

Jeffrey L. Miller, MB, BCh, FCP (SA), FACP
Associate Professor, Division of Endocrinology and Metabolism, Hahnemann University, Philadelphia

Library of Congress Cataloging-in-Publication Data

Endocrine problems.

(NurseReview)
Includes bibliographies and index.
1. Endocrine glands—Diseases.
2. Nursing.
I. Springhouse Corporation.   II. Series.
[DNLM: 1. Endocrinology—nurses' instruction.
WK 100 E5156]
RC649.E522   1987   616.4
86-23038
ISBN 0-87434-183-3 (sc)

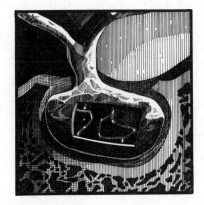

Contents

Endocrine Principles

1 Endocrine Glands and Hormones: An Overview   3

Pituitary Gland

2 Pituitary Disorders: Pituitary Tumors, Diabetes Insipidus, and Other Problems   17

Thyroid Gland

3 Thyroid Disorders: Hyperthyroidism, Hypothyroidism, and Other Problems   48

Parathyroid Glands

4 Parathyroid Disorders: Hyperparathyroidism, Hypoparathyroidism, and Other Problems   69

Pancreas

5 Pancreatic Disorders: Diabetes Mellitus and Hypoglycemia   90

Adrenal Glands

6 Adrenal Disorders: Cushing's Syndrome, Adrenocortical Insufficiency, and Other Problems   130

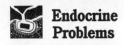
Introduction

Sometimes subtle or slowly progressive, endocrine problems often prove difficult to spot. Yet they can cause wide-ranging effects. Often, affected patients know something is wrong but display no obvious signs of injury or illness. They count on you to help identify their problem and to intervene appropriately.

Endocrine Problems helps you do just that. Written by recognized experts, it serves as an up-to-date clinical reference that reviews endocrine fundamentals, assessment, diagnostic tests, and disorders of the pituitary, thyroid, parathyroids, pancreas, and adrenal gland.

Throughout the book, you'll find information presented according to the nursing process, outlining your role every step of the way. Sample nursing care plans help you put nursing diagnoses into action by outlining patient goals, detailing nursing interventions, and specifying outcome criteria.

The book's first chapter provides an overview of endocrine glands and hormones. You'll review endocrine anatomy and function, and then take a close look at the causes of endocrine problems. One chart outlines common signs and symptoms; another presents laboratory findings that suggest endocrine disorders. The text discusses your role in patient education and promoting compliance with treatment.

The next chapter covers the pituitary gland. You'll review pituitary structure and function, including a detailed listing of pituitary hormones. Pituitary disorders often develop gradually and present wide-ranging signs and symptoms, so the text provides sample questions to ask and specific signs to look for to help focus your assessment. Selected laboratory tests, their purpose, and nursing considerations are covered in a two-page chart.

The chapter then describes pituitary tumors and their effects. You'll review hyperpituitarism and hypopituitarism. The text offers guidance on ways to educate the patient and relieve his anxiety about surgery, radiation, and other measures. You'll also take a look at diabetes inspidus and other disorders.

The next chapter addresses the thyroid gland and thyroid disorders. The text reviews thyroid gland structure, thyroid hormone regulation, and the thyroid's effect on essential body functions. You'll learn about specific signs of thyroid disorders that you can spot during the physical examination. Laboratory tests, so crucial to diagnosing these disorders, are discussed in depth, along with nursing considerations and test implications.

Next, you'll take a close look at hyperthyroidism. Physical signs are illustrated, and a checklist helps you to intervene during thyroid storm. Patients who undergo thyroid surgery will benefit from your postoperative care, outlined in the text. The chapter also discusses hypothyroidism, showing its signs and symptoms, detailing drug therapies, and reviewing your role in patient teaching and long-term management.

The "Parathyroid Disorders" chapter addresses the functions of the tiny parathyroid glands. You'll review the interrelation of parathyroid hormones, calcium, and phosphate and selected laboratory tests

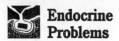
Introduction

that indicate an imbalance. A diagram helps you recognize key signs and symptoms that may appear in other body systems. Your postoperative role is clearly defined, as are interventions other than surgery.

The chapter on pancreatic disorders focuses on diabetes mellitus, the best-known endocrine problem. You'll review pancreatic function and hormones and the complex way they affect metabolism. The text looks at the pathophysiology of diabetes and ways you can recognize signs of the disease.

To avoid the devastating consequences of uncontrolled diabetes, you must help the patient comply with insulin therapy (if indicated), modify his diet, and initiate an exercise program. The chapter assists you with practical, proven tips. You'll also review blood glucose monitoring methods so that you can train the patient in self-monitoring. The text outlines other self-care techniques you can teach the patient. It also reviews signs and symptoms of diabetic ketoacidosis and emergency nursing interventions.

The final chapter covers adrenal disorders, which present a particular challenge to your assessment skills. Although these disorders often cause signs and symptoms that mimic other illnesses, a delayed diagnosis could be fatal. The text emphasizes physical signs that may alert you and provides an in-depth explanation of adrenocortical function tests.

Cushing's syndrome is discussed, along with a clearly labeled diagram indicating its physical signs. The text details nursing priorities and major complications of the syndrome. Addison's disease is also reviewed. The chapter emphasizes your all-important role as patient educator and emotional supporter during the disease's long, relentless course.

Concluding with references and an index, **Endocrine Problems** promises to be an important and practical addition to your nursing library. Like all the other volumes in the NurseReview series, it provides a professional boost in today's challenging health care environment.

Endocrine Glands and Hormones: An Overview

Marlene M. Ciranowicz, who wrote this chapter, is an Independent Nursing Consultant. She received her BSN from Gwynedd Mercy College, Gwynedd Valley, Pa., and her MSN from the University of Pennsylvania, Philadelphia.

The endocrine system helps maintain homeostasis by regulating the hundreds of chemical reactions involved in growth, maturation, reproduction, metabolism, and even behavior. To skillfully assess and care for a patient with an endocrine problem, you'll need to be thoroughly familiar with endocrine anatomy and physiology. In this chapter, we'll review these fundamentals. In later chapters, we'll give detailed information on specific endocrine gland functions and disorders.

Because the endocrine system's so complex, we'll review only those endocrine hormones and disorders associated with the pituitary gland, thyroid gland, parathyroid glands, adrenal glands, and pancreas.

Major endocrine components include *glands,* specialized cell clusters, and *hormones,* substances secreted by glands in response to nervous system stimulation.

Because endocrine glands release their hormones directly into the bloodstream rather than through ducts, they're called ductless glands. Blood carries hormones to specific cells or organs, known as target sites, where each hormone triggers certain physiologic changes. Endocrine glands include the pituitary gland, thyroid gland, parathyroid glands, adrenal glands, ovaries, and testes.

By comparison, *exocrine glands* have ducts that channel secretions to nearby tissues. Exocrine glands include sweat glands, salivary glands, lacrimal glands, the prostate gland, the stomach, and intestinal glands. The body also has *paracrine glands,* cell clusters that act on local rather than distant structures. The brain, heart, kidneys, and GI tract contain these glands.

The pancreas, unique among glands, has both endocrine and exocrine features. The islets of Langerhans, scattered throughout the pancreas, lack ducts, while surrounding pancreatic tissue contains them. (The pancreas also produces somatostatin, a hormone with paracrine effects.)

Hormone structure and function

Researchers have identified over 50 hormones, secreted from endocrine glands and other tissues, that regulate body functions. The endocrine system's functioning units, hormones exert biochemical effects on their target sites directly or indirectly, through another endocrine gland. For example, adrenocorticotropic hormone (ACTH), secreted by the pituitary gland, directly stimulates the adrenal gland, enlarging the adrenal cortex and increasing its hormonal secretions. (The suffix *-trophic* or *-tropic* in a hormone's name means the hormone stimulates another endocrine gland.) Some hormones affect target sites both directly and indirectly.

How specifically a hormone acts depends on the target cells' specific hormone receptors. However, a cell's *response* depends on its genetic programming. Thus, the same hormone may have different effects on different cells.

Besides endocrine hormones, many other chemicals travel through the bloodstream to trigger physiologic changes; however, they're not considered true hormones. Called parahormones, these chem-

Continued on page 6

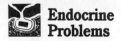
Endocrine Glands and Hormones

Reviewing endocrine anatomy

The *pituitary gland,* also known as the hypophysis, rests in the sella turcica—a sphenoid bone depression in the brain's base. Pea-sized, it measures only about ⅜" (1 cm) in diameter and weighs less than 0.75 g.

The pituitary gland has three regions. The largest, the anterior pituitary lobe (adenohypophysis), produces six hormones: somatotropin, also called growth hormone (GH); thyrotropin, or thyroid-stimulating hormone (TSH); corticotropin, or adrenocorticotropic hormone (ACTH); follicle-stimulating hormone (FSH); luteinizing hormone (LH); and mammotropin, or prolactin (PRL).

The posterior pituitary lobe (neurohypophysis), which makes up about 25% of the gland, secretes oxytocin and vasopressin (also called antidiuretic hormone [ADH]). Produced by the hypothalamus, these hormones travel down nerve endings to the posterior pituitary, where they're stored for future use.

The pars intermedia, a narrow tissue band between the anterior and posterior pituitary regions, produces only one known hormone—melanocyte-stimulating hormone (MSH). Because the pars intermedia produces ACTH in other mammals,

some experts believe it plays the same role in human beings.

Lying partially in front of the trachea, the *thyroid gland* sits directly below the larynx. Two lobes, one on either side of the trachea, join with a narrow tissue bridge called the isthmus, giving the thyroid its butterfly shape. The lobes function as one unit to produce the hormones thyroxine (T_4), triiodothyronine (T_3), and thyrocalcitonin. T_3 and T_4 also collectively go by the name thyroid hormone.

Four *parathyroid glands* lie embedded on the thyroid's posterior surface, one in each corner. A few people have only three parathyroid glands, while others have more than four. In such cases, the other parathyroid glands compensate to prevent dysfunction. Like the thyroid, the parathyroid glands work together as a single gland, producing parathormone (PTH) and small amounts of calcitonin. (Calcitonin and thyrocalcitonin—actually the same hormone—originate in different sites, with most produced by the thyroid as thyrocalcitonin.)

The two *adrenal glands,* sometimes called the suprarenal glands, sit atop the kidneys. Each contains two distinct endocrine glands with separate

Continued

Pineal gland

Parathyroid glands (on posterior thyroid surface)

Adrenal glands

Pituitary gland

Thyroid gland

Thymus

Pancreas (islets of Langerhans)

Ovaries

Endocrine Glands and Hormones

Reviewing endocrine anatomy—*Continued*

functions. The inner core, called the medulla, produces the catecholamines epinephrine and norepinephrine. Because these hormones play important roles in the autonomic nervous system, the adrenal medulla's also considered a neural structure.

The outer and much larger adrenal portion, called the cortex, has three zones. The outermost zone, the zona glomerulosa, produces mineralocorticoids—primarily aldosterone. This hormone mainly aids serum sodium and potassium regulation.

The zona fasciculata, the middle and largest zone, produces the glucocorticoids cortisol (hydrocortisone), cortisone, and corticosterone. It also produces small amounts of the sex hormones androgen and estrogen.

The inner zone, or zona reticularis, also produces glucocorticoids and sex hormones.

The *pancreas* lies across the posterior abdominal wall, in the upper left quadrant behind the stomach. The islets of Langerhans, which perform this gland's endocrine function, contain alpha, beta, and delta cells. Alpha cells produce glucagon, beta cells produce insulin, and delta cells produce

somatostatin. (The hypothalamus and the gastrointestinal tract also produce somatostatin.)

Two *testes* enclosed within the male scrotum contain interstitial cell clusters called Leydig's cells, which produce the male sex hormone testosterone.

Women have two *ovaries* in the abdominal cavity, one on either side of the uterus. Ovaries produce the estrogens estrone and estradiol as well as progesterone (from the corpus luteum).

Other hormone-producing endocrine glands have poorly understood functions. The *thymus gland,* located below the sternum, contains lymphatic tissue. Although it produces the hormones thymosin and thymopoietin, its major role seems related to the immune system because it produces T cells, important in cell-mediated immunity. Now considered an important immune structure, it's usually discussed as part of that system.

The tiny *pineal gland*—only about ¼″ (8 mm) in diameter—lies at the back of the brain's third ventricle. Although it produces the hormone melatonin, its endocrine role hasn't been clearly identified.

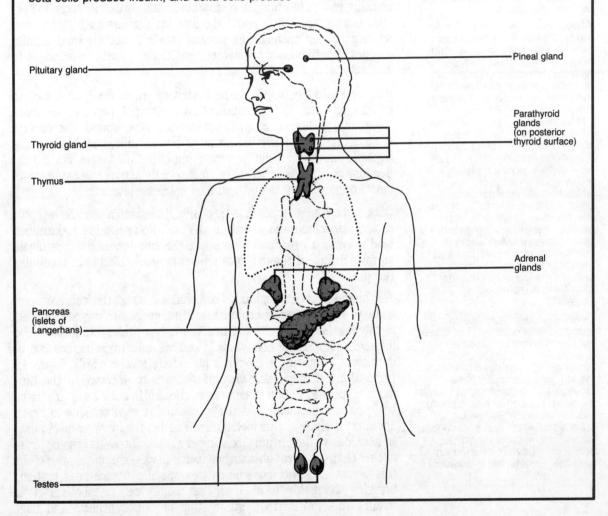

Pineal gland

Pituitary gland

Parathyroid glands (on posterior thyroid surface)

Thyroid gland

Thymus

Adrenal glands

Pancreas (islets of Langerhans)

Testes

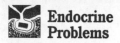
Endocrine Glands and Hormones

Atriopeptin: The heart's hormone

Scientists recently discovered atriopeptin, a peptide hormone that helps regulate renal and cardiovascular homeostasis. Stored in the heart's atrial cells, this hormone selectively but potently modifies blood pressure and fluid and electrolyte balance.

Stored as atriopeptigen, the hormone circulates as atriopeptin, acting through extracellular receptors. Directly affecting the kidneys, atriopeptin causes changes in sodium and water metabolism, such as increased glomerular filtration, natriuresis (increased urinary sodium excretion), diuresis, aldosterone inhibition, and vasopressin suppression (when vasopressin's elevated as a result of dehydration or hemorrhage).

Atriopeptin helps control blood pressure by suppressing elevated serum renin levels and relaxing blood vessels directly, thus reducing vascular resistance.

Although atriopeptin's still under study, evidence suggests that the heart's atria release small atriopeptin amounts continuously but also secrete more during atrial stretch. Basal atriopeptin levels, measured by radioimmunoassay, range from 10 to 70 pg/ml. Atriopeptin levels rise with such diseases as chronic renal failure and congestive heart failure and with conditions causing atrial stretch, for example, postural changes, saline solution infusion, use of vasoconstricting agents, high sodium intake, and atrial tachycardia. (Studies of patients with atrial tachycardia suggest atriopeptin release results from increased cardiac pressures and intravascular volume. In these patients, atriopeptin levels declined when tachycardia stopped.)

Ongoing studies continue to investigate how parenteral atriopeptin affects diuresis, vasodilation, and aldosterone inhibition. Because atriopeptin directly affects the kidney's glomeruli, it may prove useful in patients with renal injury who become insensitive to tubular diuretics. By leading to substantial water and sodium loss without marked potassium depletion, it may have a clear advantage over conventional diuretics.

Hormone structure and function—*continued*

icals include secretin, gastrin, carbon dioxide, and prostaglandins (see *Parahormones: Hormone imitators*).

Classifying hormones. A hormone's structure can be polypeptide, steroid, or amine. Proteins with a defined, genetically coded structure, *polypeptides* include anterior and posterior pituitary hormones, parathyroid hormone (parathormone), and the pancreatic hormones insulin and glucagon.

Steroids, derived from cholesterol, resemble cholesterol structurally. Examples include the adrenocortical hormones aldosterone and cortisol and the sex hormones secreted by the adrenal cortex and the gonads (ovaries and testes).

Amines, made up of selected amino acids, derive from tyrosine. They include thyroid hormones and catecholamines (epinephrine, norepinephrine, and dopamine).

Hormone release and transmission

While all hormone release results from endocrine gland stimulation, release patterns vary greatly. ACTH and cortisol—responding to body rhythm cycles—are released in irregular spurts, with levels peaking in the morning. Parathormone and prolactin secretion occurs more evenly throughout the day. Insulin has both steady and sporadic release patterns. Pancreatic beta cells secrete small insulin amounts continuously but secrete additional insulin in response to food intake.

Released into the bloodstream, hormones travel freely or bound to plasma proteins. Catecholamines and most polypeptides circulate freely; thyroid hormones and most steroids travel bound. The amount of bound steroid or thyroid hormone has significance: binding biologically inactivates the hormone, inhibiting its target-site action. Because only the free hormone's biologically active, laboratory tests must measure both bound and free hormone levels.

Once a hormone reaches its target site, it binds to a specific receptor on the cell membrane or within the cell. Polypeptides and amines bind to cell wall receptor sites while the smaller, more lipid-soluble steroids diffuse through the cell membrane and bind to intracellular receptors.

The binding process induces hormonal action at the cellular level through one of two mechanisms. Binding occurring at the cell membrane (such as with amines and polypeptides) stimulates the intracellular enzyme adenyl cyclase. This substance increases production of adenosine $3':5''$-cyclic phosphate (cyclic AMP), which, in turn, alters intracellular enzyme activity to accomplish the hormone's specific action. Because cyclic AMP acts as a mediator between the hormone and the intracellular environment to bring about rapid change, this mechanism's called the *mediator mechanism* (it activates or deactivates existing enzymes). Steroids trigger physiologic changes through another mechanism—*enzyme synthesis*. In this process, the hormone binds to a specific intracellular protein, bringing about protein changes that modify cell metabolism. As a result, DNA forms RNA, stimulating protein synthesis and triggering the change required to regulate body function and maintain

Endocrine Glands and Hormones

Parahormones: Hormone imitators

Not true hormones, parahormones trigger hormonelike effects on various organs. Some important parahormones include those described below.

Carbon dioxide
Source
Cell metabolism
Main function
Regulates respiration

Cholecystokinin
Source
Duodenal mucosa
Main function
Stimulates gallbladder to release bile

Enterogastrone
Source
Duodenal mucosa
Main function
Inhibits gastric juice secretion

Gastrin
Source
Stomach's pyloric mucosa
Main function
Stimulates gastric juice secretion

Histamine
Source
Damaged tissue
Main function
Increases capillary permeability

Prostaglandins
Source
Fatty acids in various body organs
Main functions
Increase kidney's sodium excretion, aid skin keratinization, and stimulate smooth muscle contraction

Secretin
Source
Duodenal mucosa
Main function
Stimulates pancreatic juice secretion

homeostasis. Unlike the mediator mechanism, enzyme synthesis brings about change slowly, taking up to several hours.

Hormone secretion

To maintain the body's delicate homeostatic balance, a feedback mechanism involving other hormones, blood chemicals, and the nervous system regulates hormone secretion. The term feedback reflects the return of information required to signal, or feed back, hormone levels to endocrine glands to trigger desired changes.

Hormone-to-hormone regulation. This process results from feedback from two hormonal pathways: the pituitary–target gland axis and the hypothalamic–pituitary–target gland axis.

• *Pituitary–target gland axis.* The pituitary gland regulates other endocrine glands through tropic hormones, including ACTH, thyroid-stimulating hormone (TSH), and luteinizing hormone (LH). ACTH regulates the adrenal cortex mainly through its effects on cortisol, although it may also modify aldosterone somewhat. TSH regulates the thyroid hormones thyroxine (T_4) and triiodothyronine (T_3), while LH regulates gonadal hormones. Tropic hormones get feedback about their specific target glands by continually monitoring levels of hormones produced by these glands. If a change occurs, the tropic hormone corrects it in one of two ways: by stimulating its target gland, causing an increase in both tropic and target gland hormones; or by stopping its target gland stimulation, inhibiting both tropic and target gland hormones.

A tropic hormone increases or decreases its stimulation from moment to moment by continuously monitoring its feedback and changing its own level in the direction opposite its target gland hormone. For example, if the cortisol level rises, ACTH decreases its own level to reduce adrenal cortex stimulation, which, in turn, decreases cortisol secretion. If the cortisol level drops, the ACTH level rises, stimulating the adrenal cortex to produce more cortisol.

• *Hypothalamic–pituitary–target gland axis.* The hypothalamus, in the brain's diencephalon, also produces tropic hormones. Called releasing and inhibiting factors, these hormones regulate anterior pituitary hormones. By controlling pituitary hormones, which, in turn, control target gland hormones, the hypothalamus indirectly affects target glands as well.

Hypothalamic hormones that stimulate the anterior pituitary include corticotropin releasing factor (CRF), thyrotropin releasing hormone (TRH), gonadotropin releasing hormone (GnRH), and growth hormone releasing hormone (GHRH). (Each releasing factor or hormone gets its name from the anterior pituitary hormone it regulates.)

The hypothalamus regulates anterior pituitary hormones by the same feedback mechanism the pituitary gland uses. Thus, it continuously monitors anterior pituitary target hormones and, when necessary, increases or decreases pituitary stimulation. For example, if the ACTH level drops, CRF release increases, stimulating the anterior pituitary to produce more ACTH. This, in turn, stimulates the adrenal cortex, increasing cortisol secretion. Consequently, an increased CRF level has a rippling effect. If hypothalamic stimulation stops, levels of the involved hormones decrease in the

Continued on page 8

Endocrine Glands and Hormones

Biologic need: The key to endocrine function

Hormone secretion ebbs and flows according to biologic need. To recognize this need, each endocrine gland depends on a feedback mechanism usually located within the gland's secretory cells. For normal function, each gland must contain enough appropriately programmed secretory cells to release active hormone on demand.

A secretory cell can't sense on its own when to release hormone—or how much to release. It gets this information from sensing and signaling systems that integrate many messages.

Although experts formerly considered hormone release (stimulation) an active process and lack of release (inhibition) passive, recent studies show both as active. Thus, stimulatory and inhibitory signals together actively control the rate and duration of hormone release.

Once released, the hormone travels to target cells, where a receptor molecule recognizes it and binds to it. The receptor–hormone complex then initiates target cell changes resulting in biologic effects specific to the target cell. In this way, the hormone serves as a signal molecule that interacts with its target cell to stimulate or inhibit the cell's programmed processes.

After the desired biologic effects take place, two other processes occur. First, the secretory cell recognizes that the biologic need has been fulfilled—a task requiring feedback inhibition. Then, all biochemical messages from the secretory cell, the plasma, and the target cell deteriorate fast enough so the sensing cell can obtain and act on new information.

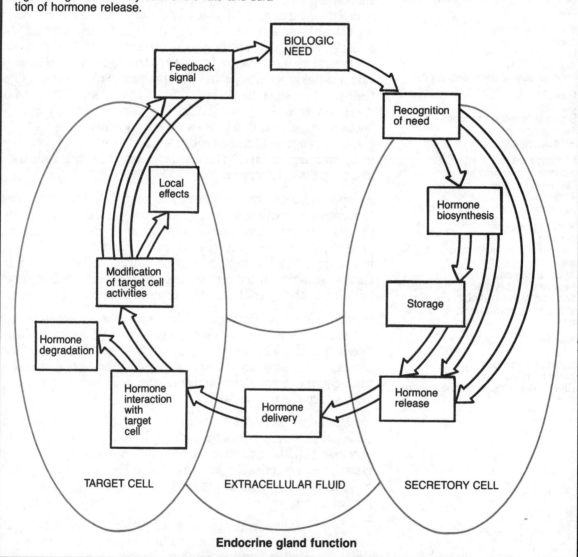

Endocrine gland function

Hormone structure and function—*continued*

same way. (For a diagram of this feedback mechanism, see *Hypothalamic–pituitary–target gland axis.*)

Chemical regulation. Endocrine glands that don't fall under pituitary control have a different regulatory system. These glands control specific chemicals that trigger increases or decreases in the hormone

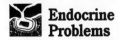
Endocrine Glands and Hormones

Tissues with endocrine features

Many tissues besides endocrine glands produce hormones. For example, the kidneys produce renin and erythropoietin; the GI mucosa produces gastrin, secretin, and cholecystokinin; the placenta produces human chorionic gonadotropin (HCG), human placental lactogen (HPL), estrogen, and progesterone. Some tumors may also produce hormones. And scientists recently found that the heart's atria secrete a hormone (see *Atriopeptin: The heart's hormone,* page 6). Because these hormones act on tissues originating within their respective systems, they're usually discussed within these other systems.

the gland secretes. For instance, serum glucose levels govern glucagon and insulin release. An elevated serum glucose level stimulates the pancreas to increase insulin secretion and suppress glucagon secretion. Likewise, a falling serum glucose level triggers increased glucagon secretion but decreased insulin secretion.

Similarly, calcium levels regulate parathormone and calcitonin (thyrocalcitonin). A calcium decrease stimulates the parathyroid glands to increase parathormone secretion, making the calcium level rise. But decreased calcium also suppresses calcitonin secretion, which prevents further calcium reduction. A calcium increase suppresses parathormone and stimulates calcitonin secretion.

Sodium and potassium regulate aldosterone in the same way. Decreased extracellular sodium and increased serum potassium stimulate the adrenal cortex to release more aldosterone, which promotes sodium retention and potassium excretion. Increased extracellular sodium and decreased serum potassium have the opposite effect.

Antidiuretic hormone (ADH) regulation occurs mainly through plasma osmolality changes, although other factors also affect ADH

Continued on page 10

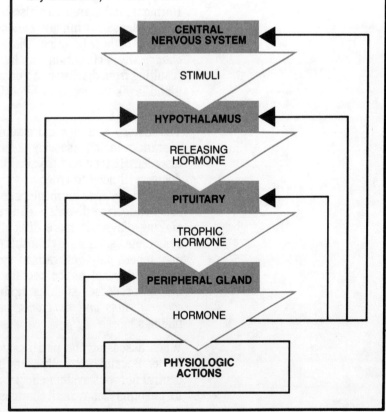

Hypothalamic–pituitary–target gland axis

As this diagram shows, information from the central nervous system travels through the hypothalamus to the pituitary gland, then flows to peripheral glands. Through the feedback mechanism (illustrated by the black arrows), the peripheral gland's hormone (or hormone-induced action) provides information on hormone levels to other endocrine glands, which then act on this information. (*Note:* Not every endocrine gland falls under each potential regulatory influence.)

CENTRAL NERVOUS SYSTEM

STIMULI

HYPOTHALAMUS

RELEASING HORMONE

PITUITARY

TROPHIC HORMONE

PERIPHERAL GLAND

HORMONE

PHYSIOLOGIC ACTIONS

Endocrine Glands and Hormones

Hormone structure and function—*continued*

levels. Increased plasma osmolality (indicating dehydration) stimulates ADH to promote water retention; decreased osmolality suppresses ADH secretion to promote diuresis.

Nervous system regulation. The central nervous system helps regulate hormone secretion in several ways. The hypothalamus controls pituitary hormones, as described earlier, as well as the adrenal medulla's catecholamine secretion. Because hypothalamic nerve cells produce the posterior pituitary hormones ADH and oxytocin, these hormones fall under direct nervous system control. Nervous system stimuli such as hypoxia, pain, stress, and certain pharmacologic agents also affect ADH levels.

The relationship between the hypothalamus and the pituitary underscores the nervous system's importance in endocrine function. Because the hypothalamus also controls the autonomic nervous system, it directly regulates epinephrine and norepinephrine—sympathetic branch hormones.

The nervous system also modifies other endocrine hormones. For example, stress, which leads to sympathetic stimulation, causes the pancreas to release insulin as part of the flight or fight reaction. The nervous and endocrine systems share additional regulatory mechanisms, but these remain poorly understood.

Endocrine dysfunction

This takes one of two forms: hyperfunction, which results in excessive hormone production, or hypofunction, which causes a hormone deficiency (see *Endocrine function: Too little or too much?*). Hormonal imbalance can also be classified according to the disease site. Disease within an endocrine gland causes *primary* hyperfunction or hypofunction. Disease in a target gland results in *secondary* hyperfunction or hypofunction. Hormonal imbalance resulting from disease in an organ or tissue other than an endocrine gland leads to *functional* hyperfunction or hypofunction.

Assessment

The history and physical examination may play a particularly important role in assessing a patient with a suspected endocrine disorder. History and physical findings may be so striking that the doctor will need to order only a few tests to confirm the diagnosis. However, because hormones affect many tissue and organ functions, some endocrine disorders can result in extremely diverse changes, making diagnosis more difficult. One patient may have localized symptoms, such as extraocular muscle weakness, while another may report only generalized symptoms, such as fatigue. Too, the patient may not notice certain changes or may attribute them to normal processes such as aging. (See *Endocrine dysfunction: Some common signs and symptoms,* page 12, for details on assessment findings.)

When assessing the patient, stay especially alert for unusual behavior. Because virtually every hormone has both direct and indirect central nervous system effects, an endocrine abnormality may lead to profound behavioral changes. Also ask the patient if he's had

Continued on page 12

Endocrine Glands and Hormones

Endocrine function: Too little or too much?

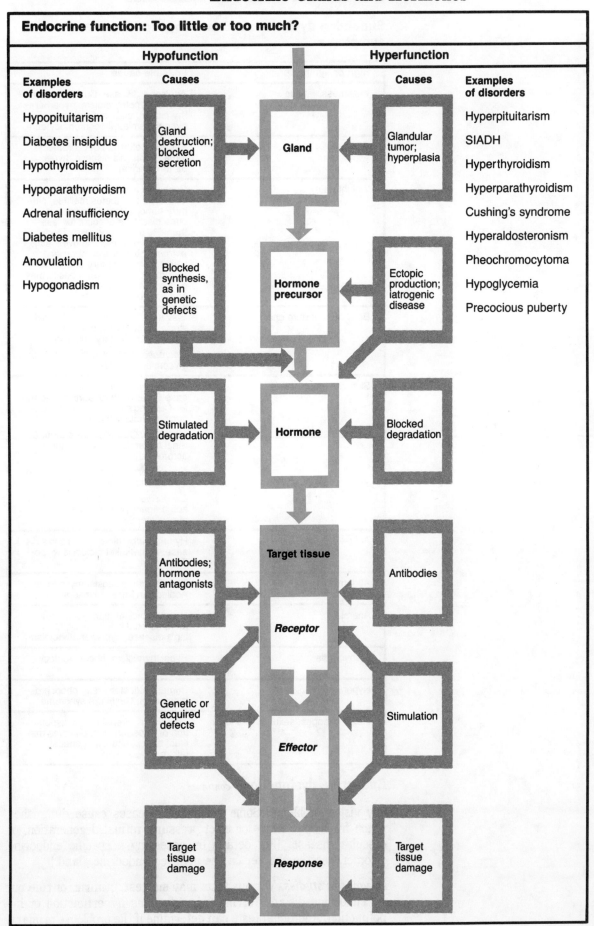

	Hypofunction		Hyperfunction	
Examples of disorders	**Causes**		**Causes**	**Examples of disorders**
Hypopituitarism	Gland destruction; blocked secretion	**Gland**	Glandular tumor; hyperplasia	Hyperpituitarism
Diabetes insipidus				SIADH
Hypothyroidism				Hyperthyroidism
Hypoparathyroidism				Hyperparathyroidism
Adrenal insufficiency				Cushing's syndrome
Diabetes mellitus	Blocked synthesis, as in genetic defects	**Hormone precursor**	Ectopic production; iatrogenic disease	Hyperaldosteronism
Anovulation				Pheochromocytoma
Hypogonadism				Hypoglycemia
				Precocious puberty
	Stimulated degradation	**Hormone**	Blocked degradation	
	Antibodies; hormone antagonists	**Target tissue** / *Receptor*	Antibodies	
	Genetic or acquired defects	*Effector*	Stimulation	
	Target tissue damage	*Response*	Target tissue damage	

Endocrine Glands and Hormones

Endocrine dysfunction: Some common signs and symptoms

Sign or symptom	Possible cause
Weakness, fatigue	Addison's disease, Cushing's syndrome, hypothyroidism, hyperparathyroidism, diabetes mellitus, hypoglycemia, pheochromocytoma
Weight loss	Hyperthyroidism, pheochromocytoma, Addison's disease, hyperparathyroidism
Weight gain	Cushing's syndrome, hypothyroidism, Type II diabetes mellitus, pituitary tumor (*Note:* Primary endocrine disorders account for less than 5% of obesity cases [body weight 30% or more above ideal]; *extreme* obesity almost never stems from a primary endocrine disturbance. However, obesity may cause various secondary endocrine and metabolic changes.)
Body temperature changes	*Elevation:* Thyrotoxicosis (thyroid storm), primary hypothalamic disease (after pituitary surgery)
	Decrease: Addison's disease, hypoglycemia, myxedemic coma
Skin changes	*Hyperpigmentation:* Addison's disease (after bilateral adrenalectomy for Cushing's disease), ACTH-producing pituitary tumor
	Hirsutism: Cushing's syndrome, adrenal hyperplasia, adrenal tumor, acromegaly
	Coarse, dry skin: Myxedema, hypoparathyroidism, acromegaly
	Excessive sweating: Thyrotoxicosis, acromegaly, pheochromocytoma, hypoglycemia
Anorexia	Hyperparathyroidism, Addison's disease, diabetic ketoacidosis, hypothyroidism
Abdominal pain	Diabetic ketoacidosis, myxedema, Addisonian crisis, thyroid storm
Anemia	Hypothyroidism, panhypopituitarism, adrenal insufficiency, Cushing's disease, hyperparathyroidism
Tachycardia	Hyperthyroidism, pheochromocytoma
Hypertension	Primary aldosteronism, pheochromocytoma, Cushing's syndrome
Libido changes, sexual dysfunction	Thyroid or adrenal cortex hypofunction or hyperfunction, diabetes mellitus, hypopituitarism, gonadal failure

Endocrine dysfunction—*continued*

any vision problems. Some endocrine diseases cause diminished vision from optic nerve or tract pressure, retinal degeneration, or vascular disease. (For details on assessing a specific endocrine disorder, see the chapter on the involved endocrine gland.)

Diagnostic studies. Various tests may suggest, confirm, or rule out an endocrine disorder or may identify it as hyperfunction or hypofunction. Additional tests can determine if the problem's primary,

Endocrine Glands and Hormones

secondary, or functional (see *Laboratory findings suggesting endocrine disorders,* page 14).

Diagnostic studies may include one or more of the following: direct testing, indirect testing, provocative testing, and radiographic studies.

Direct testing. The most common method, direct testing measures hormone levels directly as they appear in the blood and/or urine. However, because the body contains only minute hormone amounts, this method requires special techniques to ensure accurate measurement. Radioimmunoassay (RIA), the technique used to determine most hormone levels, involves incubation of blood or urine (or a urine extract) with the hormone's antibody and a radiolabeled hormone tracer. Antibody-tracer complexes can then be measured in various ways. For instance, charcoal can be used to absorb and remove the hormone not bound to the antibody to allow measurement of the remaining radiolabeled complex. The extent to which the sample hormone blocks binding can then be compared to a standard curve showing reactions with known hormone quantities. (Although the RIA method provides reliable results, it can't measure every hormone.) Because physiologic factors such as stress, diet, and body rhythms can alter circulating hormone levels, several blood samples may be obtained at different times of day.

Twenty-four hour urine testing, another direct method, measures hormones and their metabolites. Metabolite measurement helps evaluate hormones excreted in virtually undetectable amounts. The doctor most frequently orders 24-hour urine tests to confirm adrenal and gonadal disorders. The hormone or metabolite being measured determines which test technique he'll choose. When administering a 24-hour urine test, always follow proper collection procedures to ensure accurate test results.

Indirect testing. This method measures the substance a particular hormone controls—not the hormone itself. For instance, glucose measurements help evaluate insulin; calcium measurements help assess parathormone activity. (Although RIAs measure these substances directly, indirect testing's easier and less costly.)

Keep in mind that although indirectly obtained glucose levels accurately reflect insulin's effectiveness, various factors affecting calcium may alter parathormone levels. For example, because about half of calcium binds to plasma proteins, abnormal protein levels can lead to abnormal calcium levels. So, before assuming that an abnormal calcium level reflects a parathormone imbalance, be sure to rule out other possible causes.

Provocative testing. This technique helps determine an endocrine gland's reserve function when other tests show borderline hormone levels or can't pinpoint the abnormality's site. For instance, an abnormally low cortisol level may directly reflect adrenal hypofunction or indirectly reflect pituitary hypofunction.

Provocative testing works on this principle: stimulate an underactive gland and suppress an overactive gland. Thus, a provocative test may involve stimulation or suppression, depending on the patient's suspected disorder. Stimulation testing, which confirms hypofunction, uses a stimulus to increase specific hormone levels. A

Continued on page 15

Interpreting provocative test results

Hypofunction evaluation (stimulation tests)
• Normal baseline hormone level or secretion rate
• Normal stimulation test
Interpretation: Normal function

• Below-normal baseline hormone level or secretion rate
• Normal stimulation test
Interpretation: Normal function

• Below-normal baseline hormone level or secretion rate
• Nonstimulable
Interpretation: Hypofunction

• Low-normal baseline hormone level or secretion rate
• Nonstimulable
Interpretation: Impaired reserve function (may not cause signs or symptoms)

Hyperfunction evaluation (suppression tests)
• Normal baseline hormone level or secretion rate
• Normal suppression test
Interpretation: Normal function

• Above-normal baseline hormone level or secretion rate
• Normal suppression test
Interpretation: Normal function

• Above-normal baseline hormone level or secretion rate
• Nonsuppressible
Interpretation: Hyperfunction (may vary from mild to severe)

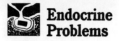
Endocrine Glands and Hormones

Laboratory findings suggesting endocrine disorders

To evaluate a patient's endocrine function, the doctor may order any of the tests listed below. For the most accurate test results, make sure your patient's properly prepared for testing and follow appropriate guidelines for sample or specimen collection and transport to the laboratory.

Test	Abnormally high levels	Abnormally low levels
ELECTROLYTES		
Calcium	• Adrenal hypofunction • Hyperparathyroidism • Hyperthyroidism	• Hypoparathyroidism • Cushing's syndrome
Chloride	• Hyperparathyroidism	• Primary hyperaldo-steronism • Adrenal hypofunction
Magnesium	• Adrenal hypofunction • Early-stage diabetic acidosis	• Hyperparathyroidism • Hyperthyroidism • Primary hyperaldo-steronism
Phosphate	• Acromegaly • Hypoparathyroidism	• Hyperparathyroidism
Potassium	• Adrenal hypofunction	• Cushing's syndrome • Primary hyperaldo-steronism
Sodium	• Cushing's syndrome • Diabetes insipidus • Hyperosmolar hyper-glycemic nonketotic coma (HHNC) • Primary hyperaldo-steronism	• Adrenal hypofunction • Chronic primary ad-renocortical insuffi-ciency
BLOOD CHEMISTRY		
Albumin	• Diabetic acidosis • Hypothyroidism	• Hyperthyroidism
Alkaline phospha-tase	• Acromegaly • Hyperparathyroidism • Hyperthyroidism	• Hypothyroidism
Bicarbonate	• Cushing's syndrome	• Adrenal hypofunction
Blood urea nitrogen (BUN)	• Adrenal hypofunction • Uncontrolled dia-betes mellitus	• Acromegaly
Cholesterol	• Hypothyroidism	• Hyperthyroidism
Creatinine	• Adrenal hypofunction • Uncontrolled dia-betes mellitus	
Glucose	• Acromegaly • Cushing's syndrome • Diabetes mellitus • Hyperpituitarism • Hyperthyroidism • Pheochromocytoma	• Adrenal hypofunction • Hypopituitarism • Hypothyroidism • Insulinoma
Lactic dehydroge-nase (LDH)	• Hypothyroidism • Severe diabetic aci-dosis	
Serum glutamic-ox-aloacetic transami-nase (SGOT)	• Hypothyroidism • Diabetic acidosis	
Total protein	• Diabetic acidosis • Hypothyroidism	• Chronic uncontrolled diabetes mellitus • Hyperthyroidism

Continued

Endocrine Glands and Hormones

Laboratory findings suggesting endocrine disorders
Continued

Test	Abnormally high levels	Abnormally low levels
HEMATOLOGY		
Hematocrit	• Adrenal hypofunction • Cushing's syndrome • Diabetic acidosis • Pheochromocytoma	
Hemoglobin	• Cushing's syndrome • Pheochromocytoma	• Ectopic ACTH syndrome • Hypopituitarism • Hypothyroidism
Red blood cells	• Pituitary tumors	• Adrenal hypofunction
White blood cells • Neutrophils • Eosinophils • Basophils • Lymphocytes	• Cushing's syndrome • Diabetic acidosis • Adrenal hypofunction • Hyperthyroidism • Anterior pituitary hypofunction • Hypothyroidism • Anterior pituitary hypofunction • Adrenal hypofunction • Hyperthyroidism	• Adrenal hypofunction • Cushing's syndrome • Diabetic acidosis • Hyperthyroidism • Cushing's syndrome • Diabetic acidosis

Endocrine dysfunction—*continued*

hormone level that doesn't increase despite stimulation confirms hypofunction. Suppression testing suppresses a stimulus known to affect the hormone in question. Hormone secretion that continues after suppression confirms hyperfunction (see *Interpreting provocative test results*, page 13, for more on these tests).

Radiographic studies. These studies, which may be done in conjunction with or after other tests, include routine X-rays, computed tomography (CT) scans, and nuclear imaging studies.

Routine X-rays help evaluate how an endocrine dysfunction affects body tissues, although they're limited because they don't reveal endocrine glands. For example, a bone X-ray, routinely ordered for a suspected parathyroid disorder, can show the effects of a calcium imbalance; a skull X-ray helps evaluate the sella turcica in a patient with a suspected pituitary tumor.

CT scans assess an endocrine gland's structure, while nuclear imaging studies help diagnose thyroid dysfunction. (For information on diagnostic tests for a specific endocrine disorder, see the relevant chapter.)

General interventions

An endocrine disorder—usually chronic—calls for lifelong treatment aimed at restoring normal endocrine function and permitting a full, relatively normal life. The doctor will order measures to regulate altered body functions and to maintain homeostasis.

Treatment goals for endocrine hypofunction can usually be accomplished with daily hormone replacement; for instance, insulin to control insulin-dependent diabetes and thyroid hormone to control thyroid hypofunction. Hormone replacement may use a purified

Continued on page 16

Endocrine Glands and Hormones

Endocrine dysfunction—*continued*

hormone (a glandular extract) or a synthetic drug that acts like the natural hormone. (The synthetic drug's usually preferred because it can be administered in a more precise dose.) A hormone deficiency may require other measures, such as an antidiabetic agent and/or dietary restrictions instead of insulin for a noninsulin-dependent diabetic. Some disorders stemming from hormone deficiency can be treated with a transplant that replaces a diseased gland.

Hyperfunction, generally harder to treat than hypofunction, may necessitate several different approaches. For hyperfunction caused by an endocrine gland tumor, the doctor may perform surgery to remove all or part of the gland. Or, he may order hormone antagonists, drugs that inhibit hormone action (examples include the thyroid hormone antagonists propylthiouracil and methimazole to correct hyperthyroidism).

Most patients with endocrine dysfunction require adjunctive treatment measures, including patient education. To help your patient and his family adapt to the life-style changes imposed by a chronic endocrine problem, teach them appropriate self-management skills. Make sure they understand his treatment regimen, and emphasize the need for compliance. Warn them that stress can exacerbate endocrine dysfunction. To help promote recovery, encourage the patient to prevent, alleviate, or rechannel stress whenever possible.

Self-Test

1. Polypeptide hormones include all of the following except:
a. epinephrine **b.** insulin **c.** parathyroid hormone **d.** ACTH

2. Stimulation testing helps detect endocrine gland:
a. hyperfunction **b.** hypofunction **c.** receptor sites **d.** binding sites

3. Treatment of endocrine gland hypofunction usually involves:
a. surgery **b.** radiation therapy **c.** hormone replacement therapy
d. hormone antagonist therapy

4. Hormone secretion may depend on all of the following except:
a. hormone-to-hormone regulation **b.** chemical regulation
c. nervous system regulation **d.** body rhythm regulation

Answers (page number shows where answer appears in text)
1. **a** (page 6)   2. **b** (page 15)   3. **c** (page 15)   4. **d** (page 7)

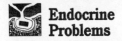
Pituitary Disorders: Pituitary Tumors, Diabetes Insipidus, and Other Problems

Linda K. Strodtman, who wrote this chapter, is a Clinical Nurse Specialist and Assistant Professor of Nursing at the University of Michigan, Ann Arbor. She received her MS from the University.

The pituitary gland (also called the hypophysis) plays a crucial role in the stimulation of other endocrine glands. Since scientists discovered its link to the hypothalamus, the pituitary has become known as an integrated component of a highly complex information relay system. Because the pituitary gland has such wide-ranging connections, a pituitary disorder can produce diverse yet subtle signs and symptoms that pose a challenge to your assessment skills. To provide effective nursing care, you'll need to understand the pituitary gland's structure and function, described below.

A pea-sized, reddish gray oval, the pituitary gland measures about ³⁄₅″ (15 mm) long and ³⁄₈″ (1 cm) in diameter and weighs less than 0.75 g. It's slightly heavier in women than in men and may double in weight during pregnancy. The gland sits in a protected saddle-shaped sphenoid bone cavity—the sella turcica—at the brain's base, directly behind the nasal base. It connects to the hypothalamus directly above it via the pituitary stalk, its major information transfer link. The optic nerves and optic chiasm also lie above the pituitary. Other nearby structures include the brain's third ventricle, sphenoid and cavernous sinuses, internal carotid arteries, and the third through sixth cranial nerves. Although this location protects the pituitary gland, it also makes the brain and other nervous system components vulnerable to damage from a pituitary disorder.

The pituitary gland has three segments:
• the anterior lobe, or adenohypophysis, which takes up about 75% of the gland
• the posterior lobe, or neurohypophysis, accounting for roughly 25%
• the intermediate lobe, or pars intermedia, which takes up less than 1%.
A small connecting strip between the anterior and posterior lobes, the pars intermedia appears well developed in the fetus but becomes vestigial in the adult. Some experts believe it's not truly a lobe but a distinct tissue type with cells dispersed throughout the anterior and posterior lobes.

The pituitary receives arterial blood from the superior, inferior, and middle hypophyseal arteries, which arise from the internal carotid arteries and interconnecting branches of the circle of Willis. A hypophyseal portal system connects the hypothalamus and anterior pituitary lobe. Anterior pituitary sinusoids receive blood from the hypophyseal portal vessels, which begin in the median hypothalamic eminence. Venous blood drains from the arteries and portal system into the cavernous sinus. This vascular system permits transport of hormone releasing factors from the hypothalamus to the anterior lobe; these factors subsequently trigger release of anterior pituitary stimulating hormones.

The posterior pituitary lobe, a nervous system extension, receives nerve fibers from the supraoptic and paraventricular nuclei of the anterior hypothalamus through the pituitary stalk. These secretory nerve fibers secrete posterior pituitary hormones manufactured in the hypothalamus. The hormones travel along the neurohypophyseal tract for storage in the posterior pituitary until needed.

Continued on page 19

Pituitary Disorders

Reviewing pituitary structure

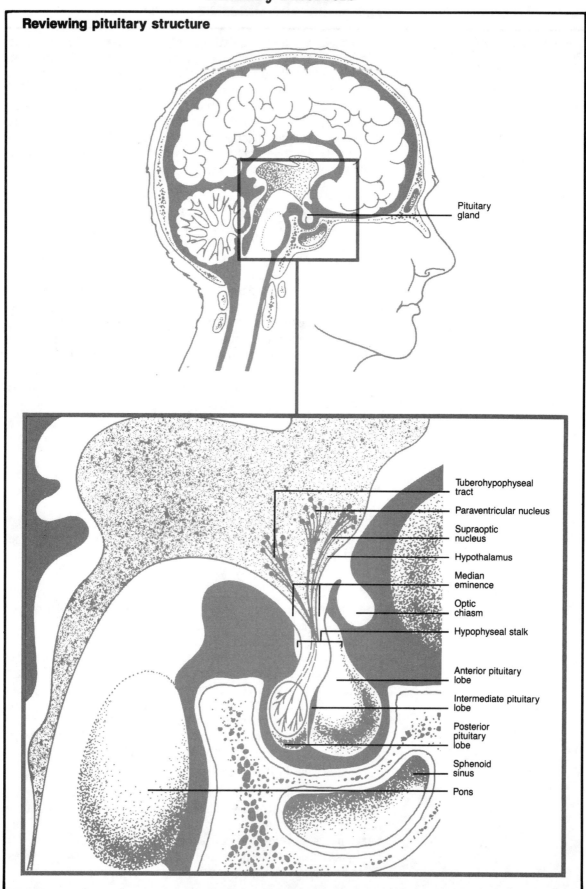

Pituitary gland

Tuberohypophyseal tract

Paraventricular nucleus

Supraoptic nucleus

Hypothalamus

Median eminence

Optic chiasm

Hypophyseal stalk

Anterior pituitary lobe

Intermediate pituitary lobe

Posterior pituitary lobe

Sphenoid sinus

Pons

Pituitary Disorders

Continued

Pituitary-hypothalamus relationship. No larger than a sugar cube, the hypothalamus rests beneath the cerebral cortex, constituting the third ventricle's floor. It regulates both autonomic nervous system and endocrine functions. The hypothalamus receives and integrates signals from nearly all nervous system sources. Its major regulatory functions include visceral and somatic reactions as well as complex behavioral and emotional reactions: temperature regulation, perspiration, GI secretion and motility, appetite and thirst regulation, blood pressure, respiration, sexual behavior, defensive reactions such as fear and rage, and regulation of basic body rhythms such as sleep and menstrual cycles.

The hypothalamus acts on messages from various nervous system sources and from vascular substances, such as nutritional factors and electrolytes. To promote the body's well-being, it transmits stimuli to both pituitary lobes, causing hormone release or inhibition appropriate to body needs.

Hypothalamic hormones that stimulate anterior pituitary hormone production fall into two categories: *releasing factors* (whose chemical structures remain unknown) and *releasing hormones* (which have known chemical structures). Both substance types cause the pituitary to release specific hormones that, in turn, act on specific target organs. Similarly, *inhibiting factors and/or hormones,* sent from the hypothalamus via the portal blood system, act on the anterior pituitary lobe to inhibit some hormones. Besides responding to body changes sensed by the nervous system, hormones take part in a chemical feedback control system that reacts to rising hormone levels produced by specific target glands. For example, when the thyroxine level increases, the hypothalamus reduces its thyrotropin-releasing hormone (TRH) output; this, in turn, causes the anterior pituitary to decrease its thyroid-stimulating hormone (TSH) output.

Anterior pituitary hormones. The anterior pituitary lobe produces growth hormone (GH), adrenocorticotropic hormone (ACTH), thyroid-stimulating hormone (TSH), follicle-stimulating hormone (FSH), luteinizing hormone (LH), and prolactin (PRL). Traveling via the bloodstream, these chemicals exert the following physiologic effects on their target tissues:

• GH promotes body growth and lipolysis, facilitates cellular amino acid uptake, and diminishes muscle glucose uptake and insulin effectiveness.
• ACTH stimulates cortisol production in the adrenal cortex.
• TSH stimulates thyroid growth and secretion.
• FSH promotes ovarian follicular growth (in women) and testicular spermatogenesis (in men).
• LH causes ovulation and hormone production by the ovary's corpus luteum (in women) and stimulates testicular interstitial cells (in men).
• PRL stimulates lactation.

Intermediate pituitary hormones. Normally, the intermediate pituitary lobe has little apparent importance in human beings. However, some scientists believe melanocyte-stimulating hormone (MSH) may form here. MSH plays an uncertain role in hyperpigmentation.

Continued on page 20

Pituitary Disorders

Pituitary hormones

Hormone	Releasing/inhibiting stimulus	Primary target site	Primary effects
ANTERIOR LOBE			
Growth hormone (GH; somatotropin)	Growth hormone-releasing hormone (GHRH)/growth hormone-inhibiting hormone (GHIH; somatostatin)	Bone, muscle, and body organs (except the brain)	• Promotes body growth • Facilitates cellular amino acid uptake (by increasing protein synthesis) • Promotes lipolysis (by decreasing protein catabolism) • Decreases glucose uptake
Adrenocorticotropic hormone (ACTH; corticotropin)	Corticotropin-releasing factor (CRF)	Adrenal cortex	• Stimulates adrenal gland to secrete glucocorticoids (cortisol), mineralocorticoids (aldosterone), and androgenic steroids • May affect pigmentation
Thyroid-stimulating hormone (TSH; thyrotropin)	Thyrotropin-releasing hormone (TRH)	Thyroid gland	• Controls thyroid hormone synthesis and secretion
Follicle-stimulating hormone (FSH)	Gonadotropin-releasing hormone (GnRH) or luteinizing hormone-releasing hormone (LHRH)	Ovaries Testes	• Oogenesis; stimulates follicle growth • Spermatogenesis; stimulates testis growth
Luteinizing hormone (LH) (formerly called interstitial cell-stimulating hormone [ICSH])	Gonadotropin-releasing hormone (GnRH) or luteinizing hormone-releasing hormone (LHRH)	Ovaries Testes	• Oogenesis and ovulation; stimulates estrogen and progesterone secretion from the ovary • Spermatogenesis; stimulates testosterone production from interstitial testes cells
Prolactin (PRL; mammotropin)	Prolactin-releasing factor (PRF)/prolactin-inhibiting factor (PIF)	Breasts	• Stimulates postpartum lactation
Melanocyte-stimulating hormone (MSH; intermedin)	Melanocyte-stimulating hormone releasing factor (MSH-RF); melanocyte-stimulating hormone inhibiting factor (MSH-IF)	Skin	• Increases skin pigmentation on exposure to sunlight (in some people) (*Note:* Controversy exists as to whether human beings secrete MSH and, if so, whether the secretion site's the anterior lobe, posterior lobe [or both], or an intermediate area.)
POSTERIOR LOBE			
Vasopressin (antidiuretic hormone; ADH)	Dehydration; decreased blood volume and cardiac output; altered osmotic pressure	Kidney arterioles, distal renal tubules	• Increased water reabsorption in distal renal tubules • Triggers arteriolar constriction
Oxytocin	Infant suckling; uterine contraction	Breasts, uterus	• Promotes lactation • Promotes uterine contraction

Continued

Posterior pituitary hormones. Produced in the hypothalamus, posterior pituitary hormones pass down nerve fibers via the pituitary stalk. These nerve fibers terminate in the posterior pituitary and secrete two hormones—oxytocin and vasopressin, also called antidiuretic hormone (ADH). Various stimuli trigger ADH and oxytocin release from the posterior pituitary, where they're stored. ADH

Pituitary Disorders

release promotes body fluid conservation and prevents diuresis; oxytocin triggers lactation and uterine muscle contraction during childbirth. (See *Pituitary hormones* for a summary of pituitary gland hormones.)

Pituitary disorders

Pituitary disorders may occur in the anterior or posterior pituitary lobe, or in both lobes. Subsequent hormonal changes and the signs and symptoms such changes cause vary considerably, depending on the disorder and the affected pituitary region.

Anterior pituitary lobe disorders fall into four groups: developmental abnormalities or congenital defects, circulatory disturbances, miscellaneous lesions, and neoplasms (such as tumors).

Developmental abnormalities and congenital defects include pituitary aplasia (congenital pituitary gland absence), which causes hypopituitarism if the infant survives; pituitary hypoplasia (a milder pituitary aplasia form); embryologic remnants (usually not clinically significant); and various anatomic variations.

Circulatory disturbances may cause such signs as hemorrhage, which may develop from traumatic head injury or a pituitary tumor. A massive hemorrhage, such as pituitary apoplexy, may result in hypopituitarism. Infarction, another circulatory disturbance, stems from decreased or absent pituitary blood flow. Usually, the patient's asymptomatic until at least half the gland's affected. With reduction of blood flow to about 60% to 75% of the gland, moderate hypopituitarism symptoms occur. A reduction to about 90% to 98% can cause severe symptoms.

Pituitary infarction may occur with diabetes mellitus, traumatic head injury, cerebrovascular lesions, elevated intracranial pressure, or severe hypoxic cerebral injury, such as from prolonged mechanical ventilation. Postpartum pituitary infarction may follow ischemia and subsequent hemorrhage and shock. Infarction affecting about 90% to 98% of the anterior pituitary can cause permanent hypopituitarism (Sheehan's syndrome). Most women with Sheehan's syndrome have total anterior hypopituitarism. Fortunately, improved obstetric care has made this syndrome less common (see *Sheehan's syndrome*, page 26).

Miscellaneous anterior pituitary lesions include acute and chronic inflammation; various granulomatous lesions from tuberculosis, syphilis, and sarcoidosis; deposition of such substances as iron (as in hemochromatosis) or calcium (associated with various pituitary tumors); or empty-sella syndrome (see *Empty-sella syndrome*, page 30).

The most common *posterior pituitary lobe* disorders include diabetes insipidus (DI) and syndrome of inappropriate antidiuretic hormone (SIADH). Primary tumors (teratomas and gliomas) and other significant lesions rarely affect this lobe. However, metastatic cancer may occur here, possibly causing DI. Other less common posterior pituitary disorders include massive leukemic cell infiltration; lymphoma; Hodgkin's disease; hemorrhage and necrosis (from traumatic head injury); postpartum pituitary necrosis; disseminated intravascular coagulation; septicemia; and various hematologic disorders.

Continued on page 22

Pituitary Disorders

Pituitary disorders—*continued*

Assessment

When assessing a patient with a known or suspected pituitary disorder, keep the following important points in mind:
• Pituitary hormones affect many body functions; consequently, a pituitary disorder may lead to extremely wide-ranging signs and symptoms.
• Many pituitary disorders develop gradually. Therefore, expect extremely subtle signs and symptoms.

Begin your assessment with the health history. This important first step helps you:
• establish rapport with the patient
• determine how his problem affects his daily life (including psychosocial functioning)
• focus on the subsequent physical examination
• guide any necessary nursing interventions.
Remember: When taking the health history, determine the patient's chief complaint, investigate his present illness and past medical history, and obtain information about his family and social history.

The patient may have various chief complaints related to endocrine function—or he may have a seemingly unrelated complaint. To elicit the patient's chief complaint, you may want to ask questions such as the following:
• Can you describe your health problem?
• When did you first notice it?
• Did it develop gradually or suddenly? (Although most pituitary problems develop slowly, pituitary trauma may cause abrupt signs and symptoms.)
• What seems to bring on the problem?
• Have you tried to treat it yourself with home remedies, over-the-counter medications, or other measures?
• Have you received any treatment from a doctor for this problem?

Pituitary disorders typically produce signs and symptoms that fall into the major categories shown on the next few pages. To help detect a pituitary disorder, investigate each category systematically by asking questions such as those we've listed. (For assessment details on specific pituitary disorders, see later pages.)

Nutritional/metabolic pattern: Do you have a strong appetite or feel unusually hungry? Have you had any nausea or vomiting? Do you strongly prefer certain foods or fluids? How much salt do you use in cooking or at the table? (Salt craving, related to decreased adrenal mineralocorticoids, may accompany hypopituitarism.) How cold do you like your beverages? How much fluid do you drink daily? Do you have unusual thirst? Does fluid intake relieve your thirst? (Preference for large volumes—up to several gallons—of ice-cold liquids may indicate diabetes insipidus. The patient may say that he can't seem to drink enough, or has to get up in the middle of the night to drink. Adding lots of ice to beverages also suggests diabetes insipidus.) Have you noticed any changes in your ability to chew food or in your mouth size? *If the patient wears dentures:* Do your dentures fit as well as they used to? (Excessive GH can alter dentition.)

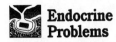
Pituitary Disorders

What's your pattern of weight gain or loss? Have you recently gained or lost weight fairly evenly throughout your body or only in certain areas? (A relatively even weight loss commonly accompanies hypopituitarism and diabetes insipidus; an uneven weight gain may mean Cushing's syndrome.)

Does your skin seem unusually dry or oily? How well do you heal after minor injuries such as cuts or bruises? Do you bruise easily? Has your skin color changed? Do you tan less easily than you used to? Does your skin look darker or paler than usual? Have any body areas lightened in color? Has your hair color, amount, or texture changed? Have you noticed any hair loss? (Skin pigmentation and hair growth changes may indicate a pituitary disorder.)

Elimination pattern: How often and how much do you urinate? Do you get up at night to urinate? Does the urine look dilute or concentrated? (Dilute urine may indicate diabetes insipidus.) Describe your bowel movement pattern. Have you had any constipation or diarrhea? (Constipation may stem from fluid loss, such as with diabetes insipidus; diarrhea may signal water intoxication. Bowel function changes may also result from thyroid hormone dysfunction, such as diminished TSH [causing constipation] or increased TSH [causing diarrhea].)

Do you perspire excessively? Do you perspire more or less than before? (Increased perspiration may stem from excessive GH, TSH, or ACTH; decreased perspiration, from deficient TSH.) What room temperature do you prefer? Do you tolerate temperature changes as well as before? (Tolerance changes suggest TSH deficiency or excess.)

Activity/exercise pattern: Do you have sufficient energy for your normal activities? Has your physical strength diminished? Can you walk up stairs without difficulty? Do you have any shortness of breath or palpitations? (This suggests TSH excess.) Do you have muscle weakness or easy fatigue? (Decreased muscle strength occurs with ACTH excess or deficiency or with GH excess.)

Perceptual/cognitive pattern: Has your vision changed? Have you lost any peripheral vision or noticed any double vision in one or both eyes? Does sunlight bother your eyes? (Vision changes may indicate a pituitary tumor; peripheral vision impairment [tunnel vision] can result from optic chiasm compression.) Has your memory or concentration span decreased? Has your voice or speech ability changed? (These symptoms suggest increased GH.)

Comfort pattern: Do you have frequent headaches? If so, how often? Describe their intensity, location, duration, and any precipitating factors. (Headaches from a pituitary tumor usually occur frontally or bitemporally.) Do you take anything for the headaches? If so, does it bring relief? Have you had any joint pain or numbness or tingling in your arms or legs? (These symptoms may mean increased ACTH or GH.)

Self-perception/self-concept pattern: Have your appearance or clothing sizes changed (including hats, gloves, rings, or shoes)? (These changes may stem from increased GH.) How would you describe yourself? Easygoing? Quick to anger? Do you ever feel depressed? Anxious? Fearful? (If possible, ask family members if the patient's

Continued on page 24

Pituitary Disorders

Pituitary disorders—*continued*

had any personality change, which may signal a pituitary-hypo-thalamic lesion or injury.)

Sexuality/reproductive pattern: As a child, did you grow normally? When did you begin puberty? Has your libido increased or decreased recently? *For a woman:* At what age did menses start? Do you have

---

Menstrual hormones

When assessing a woman for possible pituitary dysfunction, be sure to ask about any menstrual problems. Such problems may stem from abnormal levels of luteinizing hormone (LH) or follicle-stimulating hormone (FSH), secreted by the pituitary gland. Here's how hormones regulate the menstrual cycle:

During childhood, small amounts of ovarian estrogen inhibit production of LH and FSH. During puberty, inhibitory effects decline, thus stimulating production of LH, FSH, and ovarian hormones (estrogen, progesterone, and androgens).

At this time, the menstrual cycle begins. The average cycle is 28 days, but it may range from 20 to 45 days.

Follicular growth and ovulation. The cycle begins with the onset of menses, when low levels of estrogen and progesterone trigger a rise in FSH levels and LH levels. FSH and LH stimulate development of a primary follicle, which secretes estrogen. As a result, the endometrium thickens, and increased estrogen causes a midcycle surge in

LH and a lesser surge in FSH. Stimulated by LH and FSH, the follicle swells, estrogen levels fall, and progesterone levels rise. Then ovulation occurs.

Following expulsion of the ovum, the remaining granulosa cells undergo physical and chemical change (luteinization) to form the corpus luteum, which secretes large amounts of progesterone and estrogen. Progesterone causes swelling and secretory development of the endometrium. Also, increased estrogen and progesterone cause decreased FSH and LH secretion. If fertilization doesn't occur, the corpus luteum degenerates, reducing levels of estrogen and progesterone. Menstruation occurs and the cycle repeats.

Between ages 40 and 50, menstrual cycles may become irregular, anovulation may occur, and estrogen and progesterone levels diminish. The number of primordial follicles falls to zero, and LH and FSH levels rise since estrogen no longer inhibits their production. Progesterone production becomes essentially nonexistent.

	Primary follicle	Growing follicle	Ovulation	Development of corpus luteum	Degenerating corpus luteum; new primary follicle
Follicular cycle					
Follicle-stimulating hormone					
Luteinizing hormone					
Estrogen					
Progesterone					
Endometrium					
DAYS	1 2 3 4 5	6 7 8 9 10 11 12 13 14	15 16 17 18 19 20 21 22 23 24 25 26 27 28		1 2 3 4 5
	Menstruation	Proliferation	Ovulation	Secretion	Menstruation

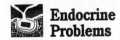
Pituitary Disorders

regular menstrual cycles? Have you ever temporarily stopped menstruating (not including pregnancy)? How many pregnancies have you had? Have you had any trouble getting pregnant or any problems during or after pregnancy? Did you nurse your children? If so, did your milk flow normally? Did you have any problems when you stopped nursing? After you stopped, did your milk dry up right away? Have you had any other breast drainage or discharge? If so, how much? What does it look like? *For a man:* Have you had any sexual dysfunction, such as difficulty in attaining or maintaining an erection? Has your facial or body hair growth pattern changed? Do you notice any unusual breast tissue development? Have you had any infertility problems? (Any of these problems may indicate abnormal GH, PRL, FSH, LH, and/or ACTH secretion.)

Physical examination. Although you can't examine the pituitary gland itself by inspection, palpation, percussion, or auscultation, you can assess its function by evaluating the patient's general appearance. To elicit information about pituitary function, observe him from head to toe. Pay particular attention to his head and facial features; posture, gait, and body movements; stature and physique; and integumentary system.

Head and facial features. Beginning at the top of the head, inspect the patient's hair. Coarse, brittle, and thinning scalp hair and lateral aspects of the eyebrows' ends may indicate decreased TSH. Baldness, thinning hair, or hairline recession in a woman may signal adrenocortical androgen excess (from increased ACTH). Facial hirsutism, acne, and excessively oily skin also suggest increased ACTH or GH.

Note the patient's facial shape. "Moon face"—a rounded shape with preauricular fullness—and a reddish complexion over the cheeks (from skin thinning) suggests excessive ACTH. Puffiness, particularly of the eyelids, may result from decreased TSH (myxedema).

If possible, compare the patient's appearance to earlier photographs to help detect any recent facial feature coarsening. Look for facial and frontal bone protrusion, nose enlargement, and overbite involving the lower incisors (all signs of excessive GH, such as acromegaly).

Note the patient's speech. With acromegaly, the voice becomes husky and the speech dysarthric (from excessive tongue and facial structure growth). The lips may also thicken. Speech may become slow and the voice may deepen with decreased TSH.

Examine the patient's mouth. Mucous membranes that appear dry from dehydration suggest diminished ADH. Excess space between teeth and lower incisor overbite suggest increased GH.

Posture, gait, and body movements. Sluggish tendon reflexes may signal diminished TSH. Bone tenderness, musculoskeletal pain, and muscle atrophy may occur with elevated ACTH. Ask the patient to squat, then rise to a standing position without assistance or physical support. A patient with excessive ACTH typically can't do this.

Stature and physique. Measure and record the patient's height and weight. Ask about his childhood growth pattern. An abnormal

Continued on page 26

Pituitary Disorders

Sheehan's syndrome

Sheehan's syndrome—postpartum pituitary gland necrosis—results from hypotension caused by hemorrhage in the hypothalamic-pituitary circulation. Ischemia and thrombosis result. This rare syndrome (1 case in every 10,000 deliveries) typically remains confined to the anterior pituitary lobe (the posterior lobe depends less on portal vessels).

Common assessment findings in Sheehan's syndrome include a history of blood loss or circulatory collapse during delivery, postpartum amenorrhea, absent lactation during the 1st postpartum week, decreased body hair (particularly pubic and axillary hair), and diminished pigmentation.

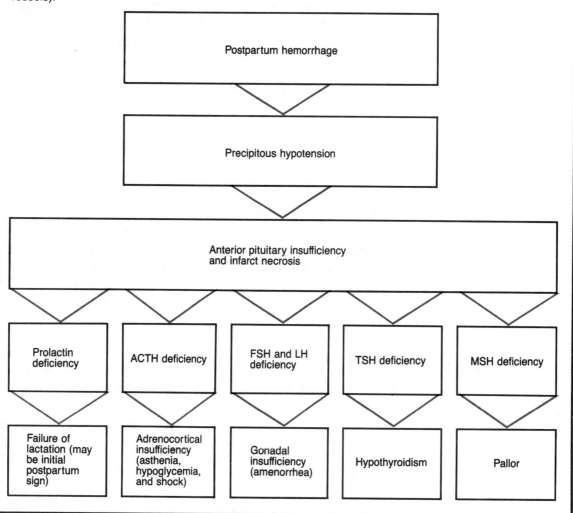

Pituitary disorders—*continued*

pattern suggests increased or decreased GH. In a younger patient, look for immature facial features and inappropriate body proportions. A perfectly proportioned body with childlike features may mean pituitary dwarfism; a normal-sized body and head with short, curved legs and arms suggests achondroplastic (nonpituitary) dwarfism. Abnormally large stature with absent or retarded sexual development suggests gigantism. In a patient over age 25 (after long-bone epiphyseal closure), check for abnormally large hands and feet, thickened heel pads, and spinal kyphosis (signs of acromegaly). Check body fat distribution—"buffalo hump" and disproportionately thin arms and legs may result from increased ACTH.

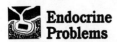
Pituitary Disorders

Palpate the abdomen for visceromegaly (increased organ size)—a possible sign of acromegaly—and palpate the thyroid gland, which may enlarge from GH, or, in some cases, TSH excess.

Integumentary system. Adrenocortical hypofunction and hypogonadism result in axillary, pubic, and scalp hair loss. LH, FSH, or PRL abnormalities may affect breast and pubic hair development. In a woman, assess the breasts for discharge, noting the color, consistency, and amount. Check for altered hair distribution, particularly a sex-related pattern, and note pubic hair distribution (however, keep in mind that racial and genetic factors also affect hair distribution).

Thick, dry, rough, scaly skin may stem from reduced TSH. Assess the patient's pigmentation. Hypopituitarism may cause depigmentation, particularly in the areolar and genital areas. The skin may appear pale, hairless, smooth, and dry. Diminished MSH reduces tanning ability. Inspect the back of the patient's hand for thinning, easily bruised skin—possible signs of excessive ACTH. Purple striae (not the pink or white striae associated with obesity or pregnancy) on the abdomen, anterior and posterior axillary folds, breasts, and sides of the buttocks and thighs may also indicate excessive ACTH.

Vision. Check for visual field disturbances. Bitemporal hemianopia may indicate a pituitary tumor (see *How a pituitary tumor can cause visual field loss*).

Continued on page 28

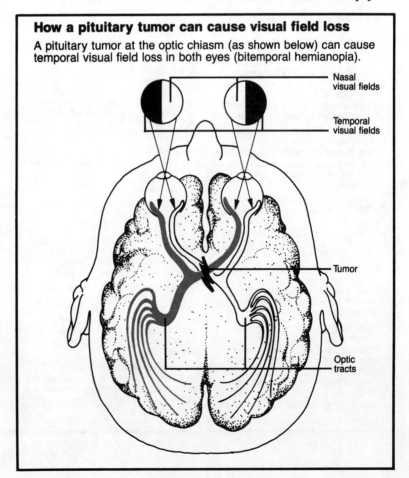

How a pituitary tumor can cause visual field loss

A pituitary tumor at the optic chiasm (as shown below) can cause temporal visual field loss in both eyes (bitemporal hemianopia).

Nasal visual fields

Temporal visual fields

Tumor

Optic tracts

Pituitary Disorders

Pituitary disorders—continued

Diagnostic studies. Two major study types help diagnose pituitary disorders:

- radiologic tests—X-rays, motion tomography (polytomography), computed tomography (CT) scans, and, less commonly, arteriography (cisternography or pneumoencephalography)
- blood tests—plasma hormone measurements, directly or by provocative testing using hormone stimulation or suppression. Stim-

---

Selected laboratory tests

ANTERIOR LOBE HORMONES

Adrenocorticotropic hormone (ACTH)
● *Serum ACTH*
Measures serum ACTH level to help diagnose primary and secondary adrenal hypofunction and Cushing's syndrome, and monitors ACTH replacement therapy

Implications of abnormal results:
Above-normal level may indicate primary adrenal hypofunction (Addison's disease); below-normal level may indicate secondary adrenal hypofunction caused by pituitary or hypothalamic dysfunction.

Nursing considerations:
● ACTH levels vary diurnally, peaking in the morning.
● Patient should relax in a recumbent position for at least 30 minutes before test.
● Alcohol intake and use of such drugs as corticosteroids, estrogens, and amphetamines may affect test results.

Thyroid-stimulating hormone (TSH)
● *Serum TSH*
Assesses for hypothyroidism and hypothalamic or pituitary dysfunction

Implications of abnormal results:
Above-normal level suggests primary hypothyroidism; below-normal level suggests hypothalamic or pituitary disease, Graves' disease, or thyroiditis.

Nursing considerations:
● TSH levels vary diurnally, peaking in the morning.
● The doctor usually orders this test only for a patient with an abnormally low serum thyroxine level.

● *Thyrotropin-releasing hormone (TRH) challenge*
Assesses hypothalamic or pituitary disease by stimulating TSH with thyrotropin-releasing hormone (TRH)

Implications of abnormal results:
Hypothyroidism resulting from hypothalamic deficiency yields a normal response; primary hypothyroidism leads to an exaggerated response. Primary hyperthyroidism and hypothyroidism resulting from pituitary deficiency lead to an inadequate re-

sponse or no response.

Nursing considerations:
● TSH measurements take place before and just after stimulation with TRH (using I.V. protirelin [Thypinone])—usually immediately, and then 15, 30, 45, and 60 minutes later.
● Test is usually performed in the morning because TRH levels vary diurnally.
● Monitor patient for adverse TRH effects, such as nausea, flushing, dizziness, peculiar taste, and urinary urgency. These effects usually last only a few minutes and may be reduced by injecting Thypinone slowly.

Gonadotropins
● *Serum follicle-stimulating hormone (FSH)*
Helps diagnose infertility and menstrual disorders. In conjunction with luteinizing hormone (LH), estrogen, and progesterone or testosterone levels, helps detect any pituitary insufficiency

Implications of abnormal results:
Above-normal level for age may indicate precocious puberty, ovarian failure (in women), or testicular failure (in men). Below-normal level for age may mean hypothalamic-pituitary system failure or infertility.

Nursing considerations:
● Values vary greatly, depending on age, sex, sexual development stage, and menstrual cycle phase (in women).
● Use of hormones (such as estrogens and progesterone) or phenothiazines may affect test results.

● *Serum luteinizing hormone (LH)*
Quantitative analysis; helps detect and monitor ovulation, assess for infertility, and evaluate amenorrhea

Implications of abnormal results:
Below-normal levels for age may indicate hypothalamic-pituitary failure, anovulation, amenorrhea, or hypogonadotropism. Above-normal level for age may indicate ovarian or testicular failure.

Nursing considerations:
● Serum LH level must be evaluated in conjunction with related hormone tests, such as FSH, estrogen, and testosterone levels.

● Levels vary according to age, sex, and menstrual cycle phase (in women).

● *Gonadotropin stimulation test*
Measures pituitary's ability to secrete gonadotropins after I.V. administration of gonadotropin releasing hormone (GnRH)

Implications of abnormal results:
Below-normal level in patient who doesn't respond to GnRH indicates pituitary disease.

Nursing considerations:
● After GnRH injection, serum FSH and LH samples are taken immediately and 15, 30, 60, and 120 minutes later. Peak response usually occurs at 30 minutes.
● Test requires accurate sample collection timing.

● *Clomid (clomiphene) stimulation test*
Assesses for hypothalamic or pituitary disease

Implications of abnormal results:
No response indicates hypothalamic or pituitary disease; increased FSH and LH levels after GnRH administration indicate impaired hypothalamic function. No gonadotropin response indicates pituitary abnormality.

Nursing considerations:
● Clomid blocks estrogen receptor sites on the hypothalamus. The pituitary gland interprets this as estrogen deficiency, causing subsequent FSH and LH secretion.
● Patient usually receives Clomid orally every day for 7 days. LH and FSH measurements take place on the 7th day and again 2 to 3 days later.
● Test may cause ovarian hyperstimulation and cystic ovarian changes (in women).

Growth hormone (GH)
● *Serum GH*
Helps diagnose dwarfism, acromegaly, gigantism, and pituitary tumors

Implications of abnormal results:
Above-normal level may indicate hyperpituitarism, gigantism, or acro-
Continued

Pituitary Disorders

ulation studies, which evaluate secretory reserve, help diagnose impaired pituitary reserve or hypofunction; suppression tests help diagnose pituitary hyperfunction.

For details on laboratory studies that help diagnose pituitary problems, see *Selected laboratory tests.* (*Note:* See Chapter 6 for information on tests that evaluate ACTH secretion [an index of adrenal function].)

Continued on page 30

Selected laboratory tests
Continued

Growth hormone (GH)
• *Serum GH—continued*

megaly may cause above-normal levels; below-normal level may mean pituitary dwarfism or hypopituitarism.

Nursing considerations:
• With below-normal levels, results must be confirmed by subnormal response to stimulation test.
• Patient must fast and remain at complete rest for 30 minutes before test.
• Stress, exercise, food, sleep, and use of such drugs as insulin, beta blockers, estrogens, phenothiazines, and corticosteroids may affect test results.

• GH stimulation tests
Administration of substances that stimulate GH release, such as arginine, levodopa, glucagon, or insulin; help assess for GH hypersecretion and aid in pituitary tumor diagnosis

Implications of abnormal results:
An inadequate response or no response indicates hypopituitarism.

Nursing considerations:
• Blood samples for GH are drawn at selected intervals.
• Monitor patient for adverse effects, such as hypoglycemia (with insulin administration); vertigo and nausea during the first 30 minutes (with levodopa administration); anorexia, nausea, and vomiting (with arginine administration).
• Provide food immediately after the insulin stimulation test.
• Patient must fast and limit physical activity for 10 to 12 hours before test.

• GH suppression test
Helps assess for GH hypersecretion

Implications of abnormal results:
Incomplete or absent GH suppression suggests gigantism, acromegaly, ectopic GH secretion, or Cushing's syndrome.

Nursing considerations:
• Patient must fast overnight before test.
• Patient receives oral glucose.
• Blood samples are drawn just before glucose ingestion, then 30, 60, 90, and 120 minutes later.

Prolactin
• *Serum prolactin*
Helps diagnose pituitary and hypothalamic dysfunction and evaluates secondary amenorrhea and/or galactorrhea

Implications of abnormal results:
Above-normal level may indicate pituitary tumor; below-normal level may indicate Sheehan's syndrome or empty-sella syndrome

Nursing considerations:
• Alcohol intake; use of such drugs as morphine, estrogens, and phenothiazines; and physiologic variations related to sleep or stress may affect test results.

• Prolactin secretion test
Involves TRH, metoclopramide, insulin, or chlorpromazine stimulation test; helps assess for prolactin secretion

Implications of abnormal results:
A prolactin-secreting tumor or pituitary insufficiency may cause a subnormal response.

Nursing considerations:
• Use of drugs such as alpha-methyldopa, reserpine, phenothiazines, haloperidol, metoclopramide, and estrogens may affect test results.

POSTERIOR PITUITARY LOBE HORMONES

Antidiuretic hormone (ADH)
• *Serum ADH*
Helps diagnose diabetes insipidus and syndrome of inappropriate antidiuretic hormone (SIADH)

Implications of abnormal results:
Above-normal levels may indicate dehydration, SIADH, or elevated serum osmolality; below-normal levels may indicate overhydration, diabetes insipidus, or depressed serum osmolality.

Nursing considerations:
• ADH secretion may increase at night, with an erect posture, and with pain.

• Water deprivation test
Assesses ability of hypothalamus and posterior pituitary to secrete ADH and evaluates kidney nephrons' ability to respond to ADH; helps differentiate psychogenic polydipsia from diabetes insipidus

Implications of abnormal results:
With idiopathic diabetes insipidus, urine osmolality doesn't increase significantly after water deprivation but does rise after vasopressin administration. With renal diabetes insipidus, urine osmolality decreases after water deprivation and remains unchanged or rises slightly after vasopressin administration.

Nursing considerations:
• Simultaneous urine and serum osmolality tests help diagnosis. Subnormal urine osmolality and normal or above-normal serum osmolality suggest diabetes insipidus; subnormal urine osmolality and subnormal to low-normal serum osmolality suggest psychogenic polydipsia.
• Test may also be performed as an overnight screening test.
• Weigh patient before test begins, then hourly. If his weight falls 3% to 5% below baseline, if his blood pressure drops, or if he has profound weakness or mental status changes, test should be stopped.
• In the overnight test, withhold foods and fluids after 6 p.m. until urine specific gravity measurement taken the next morning measures at least 1.020.
• Serum osmolality measurement takes place when specific gravity measures 1.020.
• In standard test, withhold foods and fluids beginning at 6 a.m. Urine volume, urine specific gravity, and urine osmolality measurements occur hourly until urine osmolality remains constant. Then, serum osmolality is measured and aqueous vasopressin (Pitressin) administered. (*Important: Don't* give Pitressin tannate.) Urine and serum osmolality measurements take place 1 hour after Pitressin administration. Normally, urine osmolality exceeds serum osmolality before and after Pitressin administration. After test ends, urine osmolality normally rises less than 5% over previous specimen.

Oxytocin
No laboratory tests performed.

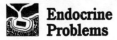
Pituitary Disorders

Pituitary disorders—*continued*

Empty-sella syndrome

Any condition causing subarachnoid space extension into the sella turcica can bring on empty-sella syndrome. The protrusion re-shapes and enlarges the sella and flattens the pituitary gland. The sella then partially fills with cerebrospinal fluid (CSF). Empty-sella syndrome may stem from congenital sellar diaphragm incompetence (as shown in the illustration below) or may occur secondary to radiation therapy, surgery, or pituitary infarction.

Empty-sella syndrome most commonly affects obese, middle-aged women with systemic hypertension and, in some cases, benign intracranial hypertension. About half the patients experience headache, which typically makes them seek medical care. However, this symptom's probably coincidental. Serious signs and symptoms rarely occur.

Anterior pituitary function tests usually prove normal, as the pituitary gland still contains sufficient amounts of all six anterior pituitary hormones.

Radiologic studies confirm empty-sella syndrome. Plain X-rays usually reveal a symmetrically enlarged sella, although any deformity may occur. (However, a plain X-ray can't differentiate an empty sella from pituitary adenoma.) Computed tomography scans noninvasively detect CSF in sellar contents.

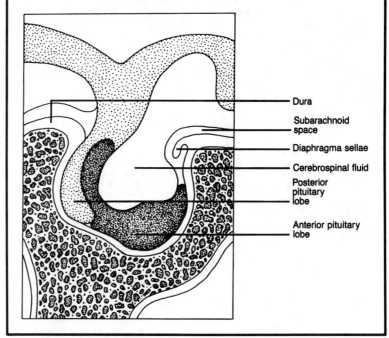

Dura

Subarachnoid space

Diaphragma sellae

Cerebrospinal fluid

Posterior pituitary lobe

Anterior pituitary lobe

Pituitary tumors

Accounting for up to 10% of all intracranial tumors, pituitary tumors may prove benign or cancerous. *Adenomas,* which constitute more than 90% of pituitary tumors, can be classified by cell type—acidophilic, chromophobe, or basophilic. They can also be classified by the associated hormone. For example, pure prolactin cell adenomas account for approximately 30% to 40% of all adenomas; GH cell and mixed adenomas, about 30%; corticotrope cell adenomas, about 8%; thyrotrope and gonadotrope cell adenomas, less than 1%; and undifferentiated adenomas, about 25%. (See *Classifying pituitary adenomas* for details.)

Pituitary Disorders

Classifying pituitary adenomas

A pituitary adenoma may contain any of the following cell types, listed below with their associated endocrine findings:

Growth hormone cell
Finding: Acromegaly or gigantism

Prolactin cell
Finding: Amenorrhea, galactorrhea, impotence

Mixed (growth hormone/prolactin) cell
Finding: Acromegaly or gigantism, with or without hyperprolactinemia

Acidophil stem cell
Finding: Hyperprolactinemia and/or acromegalic features

Corticotrope cell
Finding: Cushing's disease or Nelson's syndrome

Thyrotrope cell
Finding: Thyroid-stimulating hormone hypersecretion (possible hyperthyroidism)

Gonadotrope cell
Finding: Follicle-stimulating hormone and/or luteinizing hormone hypersecretion (may cause no signs or symptoms)

Undifferentiated cell
Finding: None

Craniopharyngiomas, almost always benign, constitute up to 5% of intracranial tumors. These tumors occur more frequently in the suprasellar region than within the sella turcica. Craniopharyngiomas produce no hormones but may cause hypopituitarism if the tumor compresses or destroys anterior pituitary tissue. The growing tumor may impair hypothalamic hormone production, release, or transport to the anterior pituitary gland. Surgical removal proves difficult, with postoperative tumor recurrence common.

A pituitary tumor can be functioning (causing hormone hypersecretion) or nonfunctioning (nonsecreting). Either type may grow rapidly or extremely slowly. A slow-growing nonfunctioning tumor may not cause signs or symptoms; a functioning tumor usually produces clinical effects regardless of its growth rate. Most pituitary tumors occur in persons aged 40 to 50.

Whether benign or cancerous, a functioning or nonfunctioning pituitary tumor may cause problems because of its location, size, and/or hormonal effects. With a functioning tumor, hormone secretion may increase. With a nonfunctioning tumor, secretion may decrease if the enlarging tumor compresses normal tissue and interferes with hormone synthesis and release. Besides effects caused by hypersecretion or hyposecretion, the patient may have signs and symptoms stemming from increased secretion of one or more hormones and decreased secretion of other hormones.

Pituitary tumors can also be classified by size: *microadenomas,* which may produce hormonal imbalances, measure less than 1 cm in diameter; *macroadenomas,* which may produce ocular and/or hormonal problems, measure more than 1 cm.

Assessment

Signs and symptoms of a pituitary tumor depend on tumor size and location. When taking the health history, stay alert for the following: frontal or orbital headache (related to pressure on the diaphragma sellae or surrounding tissues); bitemporal hemianopia or extraocular palsy (both related to optic chiasm compression), possibly progressing to optic nerve atrophy and blindness; appetite disturbance (resulting in obesity), rage behavior, altered sleep patterns (somnolence or sleep-rhythm reversal), altered consciousness (hallucinations), or disturbed temperature regulation (all related to tumor extension into the hypothalamus); diplopia or ptosis (from third cranial nerve compression); cerebrospinal rhinorrhea (from tumor extension into the sphenoid sinus).

The patient's signs and symptoms will also depend on whether he has pituitary hormone hypersecretion or hyposecretion. Hypersecretion causes signs and symptoms of *hyperpituitarism* (from a tumor and/or hyperplasia). Hyposecretion (usually from anterior pituitary hormonal tissue destruction from tumor compression or interrupted pituitary blood supply) typically causes signs and symptoms of *hypopituitarism.* Loss of both anterior and posterior pituitary lobe hormones leads to signs and symptoms of panhypopituitarism. (See *Hyperpituitarism,* page 32, and *Hypopituitarism,* page 33, for specific findings.)

Altered pituitary hormone secretion commonly causes the following changes:

Continued on page 32

Pituitary Disorders

Hyperpituitarism

Hyperpituitarism—overproduction of at least one anterior or posterior pituitary hormone—usually stems from a pituitary tumor. The pituitary gland most commonly overproduces growth hormone (GH) and prolactin (PRL), occasionally overproduces adrenocorticotropic hormone (ACTH), and rarely overproduces thyroid-stimulating hormone (TSH), luteinizing hormone (LH), or follicle-stimulating hormone (FSH). Hyperplasia—another possible cause of hyperpituitarism—may result from target gland failure or use of such drugs as phenothiazines.

Growth hormone (GH) excess

This can cause such conditions as acromegaly and gigantism. *Acromegaly* usually occurs between ages 20 and 50, after long-bone epiphyseal closure. The disorder typically has a slow onset and leads to gradual body changes. Consequently, diagnosis may come late.

Gigantism—a height exceeding 6′6″ (200 cm) in men and 6′1″ (187 cm) in women—begins in childhood before long-bone epiphyseal closure. The patient may have soft-tissue and skeletal changes similar to those resulting from acromegaly. Most die before age 30 from infection, trauma, or general progressive debilitation. However, steroid replacement and antibiotic therapy have recently improved the prognosis somewhat.

Assessment findings (acromegaly):
• abnormally wide, thick bones
• enlarged jaw and tongue, malocclusion, wide separations between teeth
• enlarged hands and feet, thickened heel pads (20 mm or more)
• prominent supraorbital ridges
• oily, rough, leathery skin; enlarged pores, excessive sweating
• excessively thick body hair
• osteoarthritis (from bone overgrowth around joints)
• hand weakness and paresthesia (from soft-tissue expansion in the carpal tunnel)
• easy fatigability
• muscle aches, joint pain
• headache and visual changes (from tumor growth that compresses optic nerve)
• libido loss, amenorrhea (in women), impotence (in men)

Assessment findings (gigantism):
• extreme height; abnormally long legs, arms, and trunk; narrow shoulders; enlarged hands and feet
• enlarged visceral organs (heart, liver, kidneys) and endocrine glands

Intervention:
• Pituitary gland removal by surgery or radiation therapy. The doctor will probably perform transsphenoidal hypophysectomy for a patient with visual impairment (unless a large tumor portion extends suprasellarly). Radiation therapy may be preferred for a patient with a smaller tumor

that doesn't impair vision; most patients achieve normal basal GH levels 2 to 3 years after radiation therapy. Radiation therapy's less likely than surgery to produce hypopituitarism; however, its full benefits may be delayed for up to 10 years.

If GH excess persists after surgery or radiation therapy, the doctor may order bromocriptine, a dopamine receptor antagonist and ergot derivative, to relieve symptoms.

Prolactin (PRL) excess (hyperprolactinemia)

This disorder (also called galactorrhea-amenorrhea syndrome in women and hypogonadism in men) usually stems from prolactinoma, a common pituitary tumor. Other causes include use of such drugs as phenothiazines, reserpine, and methyldopa; breast stimulation; hypothalamic or pituitary disease; exercise; stress; chronic renal failure; and polycystic ovarian syndrome.

Assessment findings:
• galactorrhea (inappropriate breast milk production) not associated with postpartum nursing
• amenorrhea (in women)
• reduced libido, gynecomastia, and impotence (in men)

Intervention:
• Surgical tumor removal (however, the tumor may recur). In some cases, the doctor will order radiation therapy (which has delayed benefits) and bromocriptine, to inhibit the tumor's PRL secretion.

Adrenocorticotropic hormone (ACTH) excess (Cushing's disease)

This usually results from a pituitary tumor that causes ACTH hypersecretion and subsequent bilateral adrenal hyperplasia. Hypercortisolism (Cushing's syndrome) most commonly stems from ACTH excess. Probably a primary pituitary disorder, Cushing's disease causes hypothalamic abnormalities. However, some researchers believe it results from a primary central nervous system problem involving excessive stimulation of anterior pituitary corticotropes and secondary adenoma development.

ACTH and cortisol secretion lack diurnal variation and don't respond

to stress. Glucocorticoids also have an abnormal negative feedback to ACTH secretion; GH, TSH, and gonadotropins respond subnormally to stimulation.

Assessment findings:
• obesity with central fat distribution
• moon face, florid complexion
• reduced bone mass, proximal muscle weakness
• easy bruising, purplish striae, hirsutism, acne
• poor wound healing, superficial fungal infections
• hypertension
• glucose intolerance
• gonadal dysfunction (impotence or amenorrhea)

Intervention:
• Surgical tumor removal; radiation therapy and drugs that inhibit adrenal cortisol secretion may be used adjunctively. If these therapies fail, the doctor may perform bilateral total adrenalectomy.

Thyroid-stimulating hormone (TSH) excess

This rare disorder stems from a TSH-secreting pituitary tumor.

Assessment findings:
• signs and symptoms of hyperthyroidism; for example, exophthalmos, lid lag, restlessness, irritability, anxiety, heat intolerance, tachycardia, palpitations, modest weight loss despite increased appetite

Intervention:
• Surgical tumor removal. If the patient's thyrotoxic, the doctor will order drug therapy to suppress the thyroid gland before surgery.

Gonadotropin (follicle-stimulating hormone [FSH] and luteinizing hormone [LH]) excesses

These disorders may stem from a rare gonadotropin-secreting pituitary tumor. Most of these tumors are large and hypersecrete only FSH. Pituitary enlargement may also cause gonadotropin excesses.

Assessment findings:
• depend on FSH and/or LH levels; most commonly include impotence, infertility, and visual disturbances

Intervention:
• Surgical tumor removal (drugs rarely control FSH or LH hypersecretion).

Pituitary tumors—*continued*

• *sexual functioning*—secondary amenorrhea (in women), resulting in libido loss; gradually developing hypogonadism (in men), resulting in impotence and libido loss; and galactorrhea (more common in women)

Pituitary Disorders

Hypopituitarism

This syndrome (also called pituitary insufficiency) involves deficient secretion of one or more anterior pituitary hormones. Hypopituitarism usually doesn't cause signs or symptoms until nearly all pituitary tissue's destroyed. Total loss of both anterior and posterior pituitary lobes results in panhypopituitarism, which leads to diabetes insipidus as well as typical signs and symptoms of anterior pituitary hormone loss.

Hypopituitarism may stem from a pituitary or hypothalamic tumor, ischemia (such as from postpartum hemorrhage [Sheehan's syndrome] or pituitary apoplexy), autoimmune disease, irradiation, infiltrative disease (such as hemochromatosis or sarcoidosis), infection, trauma, or surgery. The specific hormone deficiency determines the disorder's pathophysiologic process and clinical effects.

Intervention aims to eliminate the underlying cause and replace deficient hormones or hormones of affected end organs. For hypopituitarism stemming from a tumor, the doctor will remove the tumor surgically or will order radiation therapy. Nursing measures focus on helping the patient manage his self-care—particularly hormone replacement therapy, which may be complex.

Growth hormone (GH) deficiency
This disorder may stem from a congenital deficiency that slows growth shortly after birth, or from an acquired deficiency, such as from a hypothalamic-pituitary tumor, head injury, central nervous system infection, hydrocephalus, or cerebrovascular accident.

Assessment findings:
• growth retardation (dwarfism)
• fasting hypoglycemia (in a child)
• delayed wound healing (especially with bone fracture)

Intervention:
• Somatrem (Protropin) for prepubertal child with marked growth retardation (see *Somatrem: A growth booster,* page 35, for details on this drug).

Prolactin (PRL) deficiency
This disorder nearly always results from severe pituitary damage; it usually occurs only with panhypopituitarism.

Assessment finding:
• absent postpartum lactation

Intervention:
• Usually none; rarely, thyrotropin-releasing hormone (TRH) to improve postpartum milk production

Adrenocorticotropic hormone (ACTH) deficiency
This rare disorder may result from any condition that causes hypopituitarism. (*Total* ACTH deficiency's extremely rare.)

Assessment findings:
• nausea and vomiting

• anorexia
• weakness
• orthostatic hypotension
• fever
• depigmentation and reduced tanning ability
• decreased body hair
(*Note:* Except with total ACTH deficiency, signs and symptoms may arise only during stressful periods, such as from trauma or severe infection.)

Intervention:
• Glucocorticoid therapy (for example, with cortisone, hydrocortisone, or prednisone). The patient may require such drugs only during stressful periods.

Thyroid-stimulating hormone (TSH) deficiency
This rare disorder stems from reduced hypothalamic TRH secretion.

Assessment findings:
• dry, pale skin
• slow thought processes
• bradycardia
• hoarseness
• cold intolerance
• constipation
• true myxedema (rare)
• increased or decreased menstrual flow
• severe growth retardation despite treatment (in a child)

Intervention:
• Levothyroxine (If the patient also has adrenal insufficiency, the doctor will correct this problem by ordering glucocorticoid replacement therapy before beginning levothyroxine therapy.)

Gonadotropin (follicle-stimulating hormone [FSH] and luteinizing hormone [LH]) deficiency
This disorder typically involves deficiency of either FSH or LH—rarely both. Usually the result of a hypothalamic-pituitary lesion, gonadotropin deficiency may also stem from anorexia nervosa or marked obesity.

Assessment findings:
• *In women:* amenorrhea, breast atrophy, dry skin, reduced vaginal secretions (possibly leading to dyspareunia), reduced libido
• *In men:* testicular softening and shrinkage, retarded secondary sexual hair growth, decreased muscle strength, reduced libido
• *In pubertal children:* totally or partially delayed secondary sexual development
• *With isolated gonadotropin deficiency or unimpaired GH secretion:* excessive arm and leg growth from absent long-bone epiphyseal closure; may cause eunuchoid appearance

Intervention:
• *In women:* Estrogen replacement therapy (such as with ethinyl estradiol or conjugated estrogens); low-dose, long-acting androgen therapy (such as with testosterone enanthate or fluoxymesterone)
• *In men:* Testosterone replacement therapy, using long-acting testosterone preparations such as testosterone enanthate or testosterone cypionate
• *For any patient:* Clomiphene citrate or FSH-LH preparation (such as menotropins or human chorionic gonadotropin) to restore fertility

• *nutrition and metabolic status*—nausea and vomiting from secondary adrenocortical insufficiency; excessive thirst and polyuria from diabetes insipidus; hyperphagic obesity from hypothalamic disturbances; and muscle weakness, dry skin, and cold intolerance from secondary hypothyroidism

• *physical appearance*—absent growth (in children); enlarged hands and feet (from gigantism); coarsened facial and body features (from acromegaly); and plethora (reddened complexion), moon face, truncal obesity, and purplish striae (from Cushing's syndrome).

Diagnostic tests. Three major study types help evaluate a patient for a suspected pituitary tumor:

Continued on page 34

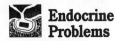
Pituitary Disorders

Acromegalic features

Common assessment findings in acromegaly (as illustrated below) include an enlarged jaw, tongue, and hands; coarsened facial features; and a prominent supraorbital ridge. Also check for oily, leathery skin; excessive sweating; hand weakness; and osteoarthritis.

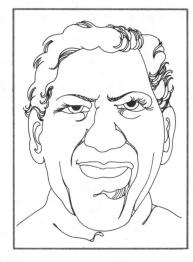
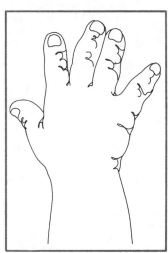

Pituitary apoplexy

A result of hemorrhage into a pituitary tumor, pituitary apoplexy occurs in 5% to 10% of patients with pituitary tumors. Typically of sudden onset, it may result from rapid adenoma growth with infarction or rupture of the tumor's thin-walled vessels. Patients with acromegaly, Cushing's disease, or Nelson's syndrome have a higher-than-average incidence of pituitary apoplexy.

Possible signs and symptoms of pituitary apoplexy include:
• a sudden, severe headache
• blurred vision
• diplopia
• blindness (from optic chiasm compression)
• eye deviation and pupil dilatation (from oculomotor nerve paralysis)
• altered mental status (possibly progressing to unconsciousness)
• nausea and vomiting
• hyperpyrexia
• nuchal rigidity.

Diagnosis comes from the patient's history and test results, which may include leukocytosis, xanthochromic or frankly bloody cerebrospinal fluid (CSF), elevated CSF pressure and protein concentration, or suprasellar extension (as shown by a computed tomography scan).

Treatment for pituitary apoplexy remains controversial but may involve corticosteroid administration. If visual deterioration continues, the doctor may evacuate the hematoma surgically to preserve vision.

Pituitary tumors—*continued*

• *radiologic studies,* which can help identify the tumor
• *laboratory tests,* which help evaluate pituitary gland function when the doctor suspects a specific hormone alteration
• *ophthalmologic studies,* such as acuity, visual field, and visual evoked response testing, which help identify suprasellar tumor extension.

Radiologic studies for pituitary evaluation include plain skull X-rays, which determine overall sella turcica size, volume, and shape; polytomography, which reveals sella turcica changes such as erosion or ballooning; head and sella turcica CT scans (with or without contrast media), which help detect suprasellar extension of an intrasellar tumor, tumor extension through the sellar floor into the sphenoid sinus, and intrasellar microadenomas; and cerebral angiography, which detects parasellar lesions, suprasellar or parasellar tumor extension, and major blood vessel involvement. (*Note:* CT scans have largely replaced polytomography and pneumoencephalography—formerly the preferred test for empty-sella syndrome.)

Planning

Before determining your nursing care plan, develop the nursing diagnosis by identifying your patient's problem or potential problem, then relating it to its cause. Possible nursing diagnoses for a patient with a pituitary tumor include:
• anxiety; related to surgery (transsphenoidal hypophysectomy)
• comfort, alteration in (headache); related to surgery sequela
• knowledge deficit; related to postoperative care
• injury, potential for (infection); related to interrupted skin integrity
• health maintenance, alteration in; related to long-term hormone replacement therapy

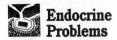
Pituitary Disorders

- injury, potential for (diabetes insipidus); related to tumor removal
- sleep pattern disturbances; related to excessive nasal drainage.

The sample care plan below shows expected outcomes, nursing interventions, and discharge planning for one nursing diagnosis listed above. However, you'll want to tailor each care plan to the patient's needs.

Intervention

The doctor may order surgery, radiation therapy, or other measures to remove the tumor and/or eliminate its undesirable hormonal effects. Nursing priorities include helping the patient cope with endocrine dysfunction and the prescribed treatments as well as preventing or alleviating unnecessary stress.

Surgery. Doctors now prefer hypophysectomy (adenomectomy) using the transsphenoidal approach for pituitary tumor removal, except for a tumor causing marked subfrontal or subtemporal extension (particularly with optic chiasm involvement). The transsphenoidal approach may preserve pituitary gland function and reduce the risk of postoperative illness and death. It also leaves no observable incision and doesn't necessitate scalp shaving (see *Transsphenoidal hypophysectomy*, page 36).

Continued on page 36

Somatrem: A growth booster

Children with growth hormone (GH) deficiencies have a new weapon on their side—somatrem (Protropin). Begun early, somatrem therapy helps such children reach normal or near-normal adult height by stimulating linear growth. Its introduction has proven especially important since researchers linked somatotropin (human growth hormone [Asellacrin]) to Jakob-Creutzfeldt disease, a fatal virus. The only other agent effective against GH deficiency, somatotropin was taken off the market in 1985.

Nursing considerations. Glucocorticoids may inhibit somatrem's effects. If your patient's receiving a glucocorticoid simultaneously with somatrem, expect the doctor to tailor glucocorticoid doses carefully. Because somatrem may cause hypothyroidism, the patient should undergo periodic thyroid function tests. If the doctor suspects a progressive intracranial lesion, he probably won't order somatrem.

Sample nursing care plan: Pituitary tumor (surgical removal)

Nursing diagnosis	Expected outcomes
Anxiety; related to surgery (transsphenoidal hypophysectomy)	The patient will: • express his concerns about surgery. • express decreased anxiety. • show he understands the care he'll receive.

Nursing interventions	Discharge planning
• Encourage patient to express his feelings about surgery. • Explain his postoperative care, including the following points: —He'll be in an intensive care unit. —He'll have nasal packing for 2 to 3 days postoperatively, necessitating mouth breathing. —He'll require a moustache dressing. —He'll need to avoid coughing, sneezing, nose blowing, and any position in which his head's below his shoulders (head of his bed will be elevated). —He'll have stitches inside the gum line (he'll feel them with his tongue but won't see them). —He'll receive frequent mouth care with mouthwashes but won't be allowed to brush his teeth for up to 2 weeks. —He'll initially have restricted fluid intake but will gradually receive ice chips, liquids, and then solid foods. —Nurse will frequently ask him about any postnasal drip and check the type and amount of nasal secretion. —He may have a dressing on some other body site (such as the arm) where a graft will have been taken to plug the operative site. —He'll have frequent urine output measurements and may receive medication if output's excessive.	• Teach patient about hormone replacement therapy, if indicated. • Warn patient to expect decreased smell and taste sensations and front tooth numbness (perhaps for as long as several months). • If patient's receiving adrenocortical hormone replacement therapy, tell him to contact his doctor if he has any illness, need for dental work, or unusual stress. • Advise patient to seek medical care for excessive urination. • Reinforce patient instructions. • Arrange for follow-up care as needed.

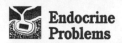
Pituitary Disorders

Transsphenoidal hypophysectomy

For a pituitary tumor confined to the sella turcica, the doctor will perform transsphenoidal hypophysectomy. The patient's placed in a semirecumbent position and given general anesthesia. The sur-geon incises the upper lip's inner aspect so he can enter the sella turcica through the sphenoid sinus to remove the tumor.

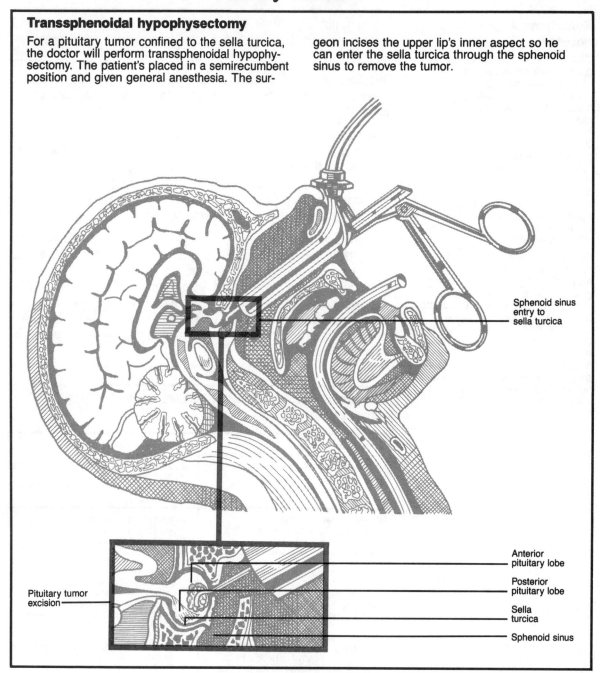

Sphenoid sinus entry to sella turcica

Anterior pituitary lobe

Posterior pituitary lobe

Sella turcica

Sphenoid sinus

Pituitary tumor excision

Pituitary tumors—*continued*

Hypopituitarism commonly follows pituitary tumor surgery. Observe the patient for diabetes insipidus, a complication of hypophysectomy (although this problem's usually transient with the transsphenoidal approach). By evaluating the patient's postoperative pituitary functioning, the doctor determines the need for hormone replacement therapy, such as steroids. (For details on postoperative care for a transsphenoidal hypophysectomy patient, see the sample care plan on page 35.)

Radiation therapy. This helps control pituitary adenoma growth or relieve signs and symptoms. The doctor may order conventional radiation therapy; accelerated proton beam therapy (cyclotron-pro-

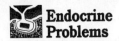
Pituitary Disorders

duced particle radiotherapy, which can focus narrowly on the pituitary and thereby avoid significant damage to surrounding tissue); or implantation of radioactive substances such as yttrium and other radionuclides (however, this may cause rhinorrhea and meningitis). Conventional radiation therapy, the most common method, has a slow onset of action and may not take full effect for up to 10 years. Consequently, this therapy may best treat a slow-growing tumor that doesn't pose an immediate threat to life.

Evaluation
Base your evaluation on the expected outcomes listed on the sample nursing care plan. To determine if the patient's improved, ask yourself the following questions:
• Does the patient understand his postoperative care plan?
• Has he expressed his fears concerning impending surgery?
• Does he appear less anxious about surgery than he did before?

The answers to these questions will help you evaluate your patient's status and the effectiveness of his care. Keep in mind that these questions stem from the sample care plan on page 35. Your questions may differ.

Diabetes insipidus

A clinical syndrome reflecting disturbed water metabolism, diabetes insipidus (DI) stems from vasopressin (ADH) deficiency caused by impeded hypothalamic ADH synthesis, release, or transport via the pituitary stalk to the posterior pituitary lobe. The causative lesion may occur in the hypothalamus, pituitary stalk, or in the posterior lobe itself.

DI can be idiopathic, renal, or psychogenic. *Idiopathic DI*—also called central, or vasopressin-sensitive DI—can stem from a suprasellar tumor, trauma (such as surgical trauma or head injury, especially a basal skull fracture), hypothalamic and/or posterior pituitary ischemia (such as from a ruptured aneurysm), infection, granulomatous disease (such as encephalitis or meningitis), or use of drugs (such as lithium carbonate and phenytoin [Dilantin]) or alcohol.

Idiopathic DI may be complete or partial, permanent or temporary. In complete DI, the hypothalamus and posterior pituitary stop synthesizing and/or releasing ADH, creating an absolute ADH deficiency. Partial DI occurs when ADH release decreases abnormally or occurs in response to altered stimuli. Permanent idiopathic DI stems from disease or injury that disrupts the hypothalamic-pituitary tract above the median eminence, obliterating ADH-synthesizing nuclei. Temporary idiopathic DI results from hypothalamic-pituitary tract disruption at the sella turcica level, with axon degeneration below. This disruption typically results from edema caused by a neurosurgical procedure. When the edema subsides, DI disappears.

Renal DI can be primary or secondary. In primary renal DI, which involves no apparent pituitary lesion, a kidney deficiency causes polyuria and secondary polydipsia. The kidneys don't respond to ADH's antidiuretic effects. Renal tubules, particularly the collecting

Continued on page 39

Pituitary Disorders

Body fluid regulation

Despite wide fluid intake variations, neurohormonal and renal mechanisms normally keep body fluid volume, composition, and concentration within narrow limits.

Neurohormonal regulation involves production, storage, and secretion of antidiuretic hormone (ADH, also called vasopressin). These processes work together in a negative feedback system (illustrated below) to help stabilize plasma osmolality. Manufactured in the hypothalamic supraoptic and paraventricular nuclei, ADH combines with neurophysin to create secretory granules. These granules, stored in terminal axons, extend from the hypothalamic nuclei to the posterior pituitary. Neurosecretory axonal fibers terminate in bulbs adjacent to capillaries in the median eminence and posterior pituitary.

After its release from posterior pituitary axonal endings, ADH passes through capillary walls into the bloodstream and eventually attaches to kidney receptor sites in the collecting ducts and on the ascending loop of Henle. In the collecting ducts, the hormone changes luminal surface water permeability; this aids luminal water transport to the medullary interstitium. In the loop of Henle, ADH triggers active chloride reabsorption and contributes to water-solute separation. These effects help concentrate urine and conserve body water. Besides acting as an antidiuretic, ADH promotes smooth muscle contraction and vasoconstriction.

Osmoreceptors, specialized hypothalamic cells, control ADH release from axonal endings. These cells detect body fluid concentration changes. Normal plasma osmolality ranges from 280 to 295 mOsm/liter. An increase of just 1% to 2% increases extracellular fluid (ECF) concentration. ECF osmolality above 295 mOsm/liter shifts water from body cells to ECF. In response to water leaving hypothalamic cells, osmoreceptors shrink and increase their electrical discharge rate; this triggers posterior pituitary nerve endings to release ADH. With ADH release comes increased water retention, and, subsequently, decreased fluid concentration. Urine concentration rises as high as 1,400 mOsm/liter. Diminished ECF concentration lowers the osmoreceptor discharge rate, which slows ADH release. ECF particles, such as glucose, urea, and ethanol, trigger osmoreceptor action by penetrating the blood-brain barrier and entering brain cells. Thus, they raise plasma osmolality but don't trigger ADH release. Sodium and mannitol, which don't cross the blood-brain barrier, raise the osmotic gradient between ECF and intracellular fluid, thus stimulating ADH release.

Besides increased plasma osmolality, other factors leading to ADH release from the posterior pituitary include the following:
• *diminished ECF volume.* Stretch receptors in the left atrium and pulmonary vessels sense reduced plasma volume (by detecting minute central blood flow shifts). Baroreceptors in the carotid arteries and aorta sense decreased volume. Less sensitive than osmoreceptors, stretch receptors and baroreceptors nonetheless yield a stronger response.
• *drug therapy.* Beta-adrenergic sympathomimetics (such as isoproterenol), narcotics, antineoplastics (such as vincristine and cyclophosphamide), chlorpropamide, and clofibrate may stimulate ADH release.
• *hyperthermia.* As body temperature rises, cells draw in more water, thereby triggering ADH release.
• *severe pain, trauma, and emotional distress.* Exactly how these factors promote ADH release remains unclear.

The body's fluid balance also depends on the thirst mechanism. Fully concentrated urine (with an osmolality between 1,200 and 1,400 mOsm/liter) activates the thirst center (located in the hypothalamic ventromedian nucleus), which then stimulates the cerebral cortex to increase fluid intake. Consequently, body fluid concentration decreases.

To evaluate a patient's fluid balance, the doctor may order serum and urine osmolality and urine gravity tests.

The *serum osmolality level* reflects the amount of dissolved particles in the serum. Electrolytes (such as sodium, chloride, calcium, and bicarbonate) and inactive substances (such as glucose and urea) affect osmolality. Normal serum osmolality ranges from 280 to 295 mOsm/liter.

Urine osmolality reveals the total number of urine particles. Normally ranging from 50 to 1,400 mOsm/liter, urine osmolality averages 500 to 800 mOsm/liter. (When urine and serum osmolality are measured simultaneously, urine osmolality's normally about four times higher.)

Urine specific gravity, which normally ranges from 1.010 to 1.030, roughly reflects the kidney's urine concentrating ability.

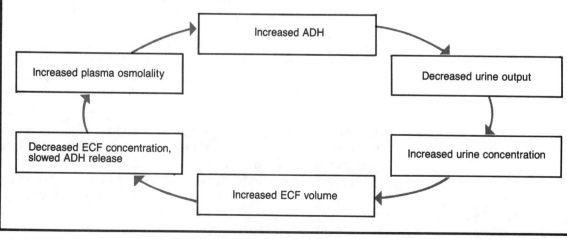

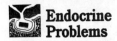
Pituitary Disorders

Diabetes insipidus—*continued*

ducts, resist ADH and don't reabsorb water. Consequently, urine concentration's inadequate despite normal ADH levels. This less common DI type tends to run in families.

Secondary (acquired) renal DI may result from:
• *intrinsic renal disease* (particularly a glomerular or vascular disorder) that severely diminishes the kidney's urine concentrating ability
• *severe protein deficiency,* which reduces urea availability (urea helps draw water from collecting ducts and concentrate urine)
• *limited sodium intake,* which causes water reabsorption from the collecting ducts
• *electrolyte imbalances,* particularly hypokalemia and hypercalcemia
• *use of drugs* such as lithium carbonate, demeclocycline (Declomycin), amphotericin B, methoxyflurane (Penthrane), and colchicine (these drugs induce diuresis by disrupting renal medullary interstitial hypertonicity).

Psychogenic DI follows a large fluid intake (usually more than 5 liters/day) that suppresses ADH. Also called psychogenic polydipsia, psychogenic DI dilutes extracellular fluid, inhibits ADH secretion, and produces diuresis.

No matter the cause or type, DI leads to water loss. Without ADH, almost no water permeates the collecting ducts, limiting water reabsorption. As the body loses free water, plasma osmolality and serum sodium levels increase. The kidneys stop conserving water, leading to reduced urine concentration. Rising plasma osmolality stimulates osmoreceptors. The normal response—increased ADH production and/or secretion—may not occur in DI, nor may the normal renal response to ADH. Although osmoreceptor stimulation doesn't correct plasma osmolality, it does intensify thirst perception via cerebral cortex activation. Thirst leads to abundant water intake, which dilutes the plasma to restore normal or near-normal osmolality. Frequent voiding also occurs.

Complications. Severe volume depletion, dehydration, hypovolemia, and hyperosmolality may complicate DI, especially if the patient has an absent or impaired thirst mechanism. A prolonged urinary flow increase may produce chronic complications, such as enlarged calyceal, ureteral, and bladder capacities. Prolonged distention thins and weakens these structures' walls.

Assessment

To detect DI early, closely monitor your patient's fluid and electrolyte status. Suspect DI if he has a urine output greater than 200 ml/hour and specific gravity less than 1.005.

Polyuria and intense thirst strongly suggest DI. In polyuria, DI's hallmark, the patient voids large urine volumes no matter his fluid intake. Urine output, which continues throughout the night, ranges from 2 to 3 liters/day with renal DI to more than 10 liters/day with idiopathic DI.

Polyuria typically has an abrupt onset. For example, with DI secondary to severe edema from head trauma or surgery, polyuria begins 1 to 2 days after injury. It gradually diminishes over the

Continued on page 40

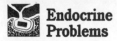
Pituitary Disorders

Diabetes insipidus—*continued*

next few days as edema decreases. With hypothalamic injury, polyuria may not appear for up to 3 days after injury, when ADH stores become depleted.

Intense thirst (polydipsia), the second most common DI symptom, represents a compensatory mechanism to maintain sufficient fluid volume. For unknown reasons, the DI patient clearly prefers ice water. Along with polyuria, polydipsia disrupts the patient's activities (including sleep), leading to inconvenience, frustration, and embarrassment.

The DI patient may also experience weight loss, fatigue, lack of energy, anorexia, and constipation from excess urine output.

Diagnostic studies. The water deprivation test (described on page 29) evaluates the patient for DI by determining whether his kidneys can concentrate urine when stimulated by ADH release. It also assesses the kidneys' reaction to exogenous ADH administration (as determined by urine osmolality).

The vasopressin test, less frequently used to evaluate DI, involves administration of aqueous vasopressin (Pitressin) in small doses over a specified period to help establish the DI type. In a patient with idiopathic or psychogenic DI, the drug reduces urine output. A patient with renal DI, however, won't respond to this test. (*Note:* The vasopressin radioimmunoassay also helps diagnose DI. However, it may not be readily available.)

Other laboratory tests that help assess DI include serum and urine osmolality, serum sodium, and urine specific gravity measurements. The DI patient with an intact thirst mechanism shows a normal serum osmolality; one with an impaired or absent thirst mechanism has an abnormally high serum osmolality. With an absent or impaired thirst mechanism, serum sodium concentrations commonly exceed 145 mEq/liter from free water loss. Urine osmolality typically drops below 300 mOsm/liter (usually measuring about 50 to 100 mOsm/liter). Also abnormally low, urine specific gravity ranges from about 1.001 to 1.005.

If the doctor suspects a pituitary tumor as DI's cause, he'll probably order visual field testing and radiologic studies (CT scans and sella turcica X-rays).

Because ADH insufficiency and resistance can complicate DI diagnosis, the doctor must rule out other possible polyuria causes, such as psychogenic polydipsia (habitual or compulsive water intake); diabetes mellitus, which leads to elevated serum and urine glucose concentrations; and chronic nephritis, which causes increased urinary albumin and, in most cases, elevated blood urea nitrogen (BUN) levels.

Planning

Before determining your nursing care plan, develop the nursing diagnosis by identifying your patient's problem or potential problem, then relating it to its cause. Possible nursing diagnoses for a patient with DI include:
- knowledge deficit; related to home care of diabetes insipidus–related polyuria
- fluid volume, alteration in (deficit); related to polyuria

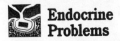
Pituitary Disorders

- nutrition, alteration in (less than body requirements); related to electrolyte imbalance
- sleep pattern disturbances; related to excessive urination
- self-concept, disturbances in; related to excessive urination
- coping, ineffective; related to disease process
- skin integrity, impairment of; related to fluid volume deficit.

The sample care plan below shows expected outcomes, nursing interventions, and discharge planning for one nursing diagnosis listed above. However, you'll want to tailor each care plan to the patient's needs.

Intervention

Treatment of DI depends on its cause and the clinical setting. Goals include maintaining fluid and electrolyte balance and identifying and correcting DI's cause. To maintain fluid balance, the doctor may order parenteral fluid administration (expect to give hypotonic fluids, as DI is usually accompanied by hypernatremia). Unless the patient's unconscious, make sure he has unrestricted access to fluids to prevent dehydration.

Also expect to administer vasopressin. If the patient has DI with a predicted short duration (for example, after head trauma or neurosurgery) or if he requires quick intervention, the doctor will probably order aqueous vasopressin. For a patient with more severe, persistent DI, the doctor may choose the longer-acting vasopressin tannate (Pitressin Tannate in Oil). See *Vasopressin replacement therapy,* page 42, for details.

When administering these preparations, stay alert for the following:
- drug resistance
- allergy to ADH or to the oily medium in Pitressin Tannate
- ADH ineffectiveness, if the patient also has hypokalemia or hypercalcemia
- vasoconstriction and angina (with large doses) in a patient with coronary artery disease
- ADH intoxication and overhydration (with excessive ADH intake).

Continued on page 42

Sample nursing care plan: Diabetes insipidus

Nursing diagnosis	Expected outcomes
Knowledge deficit; related to home care of diabetes insipidus–related polyuria	The patient will: • understand the importance of fluid monitoring. • accurately measure and record his fluid intake and output. • measure his urine specific gravity. • weigh himself daily. • know when to seek medical care.
Nursing interventions • Teach patient and family members about disease and its process. • Discuss fluid balance principles with patient. • Teach patient how to measure and record fluid intake and output. • Teach patient how to use hydrometer to measure urine specific gravity. • Instruct patient to take daily weights (at same time each morning while wearing same amount of clothing). • Teach patient about hormone replacement therapy and how to administer it.	**Discharge planning** • Reinforce treatment plan with patient and family. • If patient's receiving Pitressin Tannate in Oil, have him check each new bottle to make sure it's the right drug—*not* Aqueous Pitressin. • Reinforce fluid replacement guidelines. • Instruct patient to wear or carry medical identification listing diabetes insipidus and his treatment. • Teach patient when to seek medical attention. • Arrange for follow-up care as indicated.

Pituitary Disorders

Vasopressin replacement therapy

Drug	Nursing considerations
Vasopressin (Pitressin Synthetic, Aqueous Pitressin)	• Short-acting antidiuretic hormone preparation (effects last 2 to 8 hours); usually not ordered for long-term therapy • Commonly administered during initial postoperative period or after acute trauma • Used mainly for acute care
Vasopressin tannate (Pitressin Tannate in Oil)	• Long-acting preparation (effects last 48 to 72 hours); preferred for long-term therapy • Pitressin Tannate in Oil ampule contains brown specks (active particles) suspended in peanut oil base. Before administration, brown specks must be dispersed throughout oil. If they've settled to the bottom, warm ampule under hot water for several minutes, then roll it between your palms for about 3 minutes. Shake the ampule vigorously. Make sure the ampule's dry and that no medication's in the tip before you break it off. • Inject the drug I.M. or deep subcutaneously with a large needle, as ordered. After injection, have patient lie quietly for several minutes; observe injection site for oozing.
Lypressin (Diapid Nasal Spray)	• Used as a metered-dose spray or placed on cotton ball and inserted in nostril at bedtime (this method helps reduce nocturnal polyuria) • Provides alternative administration route • Has 1-hour onset of action; 3- to 8-hour duration • Can be used alone or in conjunction with Pitressin Tannate • Can cause chronic rhinopharyngitis and stomach upset (from swallowed medication)
Desmopressin (DDAVP)	• Synthetic analogue of arginine vasopressin • Administered by nasal insufflation, nasal spray, parenteral injection, or dropper (via dropper bottle with calibrated catheter) • Has 1-hour onset of action; 8- to 20-hour duration • Has a longer half-life and stronger antidiuretic effect than lypressin • May cause headaches

Diabetes insipidus—*continued*

The doctor may also order drugs that increase ADH's release or enhance its renal effects. For a patient with residual ADH secretory capacity, he may order a drug that promotes ADH activity, such as chlorpropamide (Diabinese), clofibrate (Atromid-S), or carbamazepine (Tegretol).

If the patient's DI stems from a posterior pituitary tumor, the doctor may remove the tumor surgically. However, keep in mind that surgery can also *cause* DI. Postoperatively, monitor the patient closely for DI development.

Pituitary Disorders

For a patient with acquired renal DI, therapy aims to correct the cause, restrict sodium and protein intake (to decrease water excretion and urinary volume), and produce diuresis, using thiazide diuretics. (Remember, the patient with acquired renal DI has ADH resistance.)

Evaluation

Base your evaluation on the expected outcomes as listed on the sample nursing care plan. To determine if the patient's improved, ask yourself the following questions:
* Can the patient accurately measure and record his fluid intake and output?
* Does he understand fluid balance principles?
* Does he know how to measure his urine specific gravity?
* Can he accurately weigh himself?
* Does he know how hormone replacement therapy works?
* Can he administer his medications correctly?
* Does he know what adverse effects his medications may cause?
* Does he know when to seek medical attention?

The answers to these questions will help you evaluate your patient's status and the effectiveness of his care. Keep in mind that these questions stem from the sample care plan on page 41. Your questions may differ.

Syndrome of inappropriate antidiuretic hormone (SIADH)

This disorder reflects excessive ADH secretion by the hypothalamus or by an extrahypothalamic, extrapituitary tumor. It's associated with plasma hypotonicity and hyponatremia stemming from irregular ADH production or prolonged inappropriate ADH secretion—secretion that persists despite normally inhibitory physiologic changes (including hypotonicity, usually the predominant ADH inhibitor). Various conditions may predispose a patient to SIADH (as described in *SIADH risk factors,* page 44).

SIADH involves a pathologic positive feedback system. Elevated ADH release persists even with increased plasma volume and decreased extracellular fluid osmolality. However, this excessive release doesn't produce fluid accumulation and edema. Instead, as the patient retains 2 to 3 liters of water, his plasma volume expands and blood pressure rises, triggering compensatory mechanisms that reduce renal sodium and water absorption. This, in turn, prevents any overall fluid gain. Compensatory mechanisms include increased glomerular filtration (which delivers a larger filtered sodium load to the proximal tubules, resulting in reduced sodium reabsorption); volume expansion (which enhances renal medullary blood flow and flushes out the hypertonic interstitium); and the natriuretic response (which inhibits aldosterone release). Thus, the patient retains water from ADH excess, then compensates by losing both sodium and water.

As a result of these compensatory mechanisms, the serum sodium level decreases significantly. Severely decreased extracellular fluid sodium concentration permits water movement into cells. In the brain, such movement causes swelling that increases intracranial pressure. Chronic hyponatremia eventually depletes brain cells of sodium, restricting intracranial pressure and volume increase. The

Continued on page 44

Pituitary Disorders

SIADH risk factors

Cancerous tumor leading to ectopic antidiuretic hormone (ADH) production (most common cause of SIADH):
- acute myeloid leukemia
- bronchogenic duodenal, pancreatic, or prostatic cancer
- Hodgkin's disease
- thymoma.

Central nervous system problems:
- brain tumor
- electroconvulsive therapy
- Guillain-Barré syndrome
- head trauma
- hemorrhage, including subarachnoid hemorrhage, subdural hematoma, and cerebrovascular accident
- hydrocephalus
- infection, including brain abscess, encephalitis, and meningitis
- seizures.

Cigarette smoking

Drug use:
- carbamazepine
- chlorpropamide
- clofibrate
- cyclophosphamide
- isoproterenol
- morphine
- oxytocin
- phenothiazines
- prostaglandins
- thiazide diuretics
- tricyclic antidepressants
- vasopressin
- vincristine.

Endocrine disorders:
- adrenal insufficiency
- myxedema
- pituitary insufficiency.

Positive-pressure ventilation therapy

Psychosis

Pulmonary disorders:
- asthma
- chronic obstructive pulmonary disease
- cystic fibrosis
- pneumonia
- pneumothorax
- tuberculosis.

What happens in SIADH

Excessive antidiuretic hormone (ADH) secretion increases renal tubule permeability, promoting water retention. As extracellular fluid volume expands, plasma osmolality falls. The glomerular filtration rate (GFR) rises, and aldosterone secretion decreases, eventually causing hyponatremia.

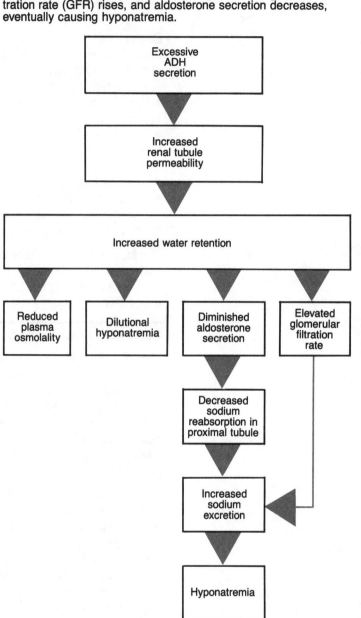

Syndrome of inappropriate antidiuretic hormone—*continued*

patient also has elevated urine osmolality. The kidneys excrete abundant sodium in the urine (because of reduced aldosterone); however, elevated ADH levels cause continued water retention.

SIADH complications include water intoxication and overhydration. Water intoxication and subsequent cell death may follow rapid-onset or severe SIADH or excessive fluid intake after vasopressin administration. (For this reason, warn the DI patient to decrease his fluid intake after vasopressin administration.)

Pituitary Disorders

Water intoxication first appears as a changed level of consciousness. Other signs and symptoms include malaise, nausea, asthenia, and oliguria. Laboratory findings reveal diluted plasma with low serum sodium, potassium, and chloride levels.

Assessment

Signs and symptoms of SIADH stem from excessive water retention and water intoxication (with *severe* SIADH). Therefore, make sure to include the following when assessing a patient with known or suspected SIADH:

• *fluid and electrolyte status.* Check urine volume, specific gravity, and body weight, and ask about muscle cramps.
• *cardiovascular status.* Check heart rate and blood pressure.
• *GI status.* Ask about any anorexia, nausea, vomiting, or bowel problems.
• *neurologic status.* Check level of consciousness.
• *psychological status.* Check for irritability or hostility.

Specific SIADH findings vary with the disorder's length of onset and severity. Gradual onset over several days causes mild signs and symptoms, such as lethargy, sleepiness, mental confusion, headache, muscle cramps, anorexia, and weight gain. Rapid SIADH onset can produce moderate to severe effects, such as personality changes, hostility, irritability, disorientation, nausea and/or vomiting, diarrhea, abdominal cramps, weakness, sluggish deep tendon reflexes, seizures, coma, and death.

Diagnostic studies. The following laboratory findings suggest SIADH:

• serum sodium usually below 130 mEq/liter
• serum osmolality usually below 275 mOsm/liter
• urine osmolality usually above 900 mOsm/liter
• urine sodium inappropriately high compared to the low serum sodium level.

Other findings that help diagnose SIADH include dilutional hypokalemia and hypocalcemia, normal BUN and creatinine levels, decreased urinary aldosterone levels, and normal thyroid and adrenocortical hormone levels.

Planning

Before determining your nursing care plan, develop the nursing diagnosis by identifying your patient's problem or potential problem, then relating it to its cause. Possible nursing diagnoses for a patient with SIADH include:

• fluid volume, alteration in (excess); related to excessive water retention
• bowel movements, alteration in (constipation); related to fluid volume alteration
• knowledge deficit; related to newly diagnosed disease
• thought processes, alteration in (impaired); related to cerebral edema.

The sample care plan on page 46 shows expected outcomes, nursing interventions, and discharge planning for one nursing diagnosis

Continued on page 46

Fluid loss: Normal amounts and routes

Fluid balance depends on an integrated system that precisely regulates fluid intake (through thirst mechanisms) and output (through vasopressin secretion). The average person loses—and must take in—approximately 2.5 to 3 liters of fluid daily. Foods or oxidative metabolism provide roughly 1.2 liters; water and other beverages provide the rest. Normally, the body's fluid level varies no more than 1% to 2%.

Fluid loss route	Liters/24 hrs (average)
Urine	1.5
Skin (perspiration)	0.6
Lungs (respiration)	0.4
Feces	0.1

Pituitary Disorders

Assessing fluid balance

Any patient can suffer fluid imbalance. Stay especially alert for this problem when caring for an infant, a young child, an elderly patient, and anyone with reduced or absent thirst sensation.

To help prevent fluid imbalance, ask the patient about his normal drinking and voiding patterns, his estimated daily fluid intake and output, his weight stability, and his medication history.

During your nursing care, be sure to document his fluid intake and output and weigh him daily—at the same time, on the same scale.

During the physical examination, check for the following indications of fluid imbalance:
• *blood pressure changes.* With dehydration, blood pressure drops and orthostatic hypotension may develop. With overhydration or water intoxication, blood pressure rises until the heart can't pump effectively; then, blood pressure drops and venous congestion occurs.
• *pulse rate changes.* A weak, rapid, thready pulse signals dehydration. A full, bounding pulse suggests overhydration.
• *level of consciousness changes.* Confusion, disorientation, and lethargy accompany overhydration. A markedly reduced level of consciousness may accompany severe dehydration.
• *muscle tone and reflex changes.* Muscle weakness and decreased deep tendon reflexes may follow overhydration and hyponatremia.
• *gastrointestinal (GI) changes.* Overhydration and hyponatremia impair GI motility, causing decreased bowel sounds. (With dehydration, bowel sounds usually remain normal unless compensatory sympathetic nervous system mechanisms reduce peristalsis.)
• *urine output changes.* Dehydration reduces urine output; overhydration increases it.
• *respiratory changes.* Adventitious lung sounds (rhonchi, wheezes, and crackles) may occur with overhydration (from excess body fluid). Dehydration causes thick, tenacious secretions; overhydration leads to copious liquid secretions.
• *integumentary changes.* Moist skin may signal overhydration; dry, scaly skin and poor skin turgor may mean dehydration.

Sample nursing care plan: SIADH

Nursing diagnosis	Expected outcomes
Fluid volume, alteration in (excess); related to excessive water retention	The patient will: • maintain fluid intake equal to urinary output (or as indicated). • maintain normal urine specific gravity. • maintain normal weight. • lack signs and symptoms of cerebral edema, such as mental status change.
Nursing interventions • Maintain strict intake and output measurements; notify doctor if fluid imbalance occurs. • Assess for urine specific gravity trends. • Teach patient about need for strict fluid intake regulation. • Teach patient about fluid amounts in foods. • Take daily weights; assess for weight trends. • Assess for level of consciousness trends; notify doctor of any changes.	**Discharge planning** • Reinforce treatment plan with patient and family. • Advise patient when to seek medical care. • Arrange for follow-up care as indicated. • Discuss with patient how to maintain fluid balance at home. • Advise patient to continue taking daily weights and monitoring fluid intake and output at home, if indicated. • Tell patient to decrease fluid intake after administering vasopressin replacement therapy (if needed).

Syndrome of inappropriate antidiuretic hormone—*continued*

listed on page 45. However, you'll want to tailor each care plan to the patient's needs.

Interventions

Treatment priorities include early SIADH detection and prompt correction. Medical intervention treats the underlying disease (or its cause) or corrects excessive water retention. For example, drug withdrawal usually corrects drug-related SIADH. Treatment of excessive water retention depends on the problem's severity and duration. In mild cases, fluid restriction (for example, to no more than insensible losses) usually corrects the situation. In acute cases (those involving abnormally low serum sodium concentrations or severe neurologic signs and symptoms), the doctor may order a potent loop diuretic, such as furosemide (Lasix), then hypertonic saline solution (3% NaCl) infusion. Furosemide (1 mg/kg I.V.) lowers tubular sodium reabsorption, which, in turn, reduces urinary sodium and water excretion. Sodium replacement with hypertonic saline solution produces a net loss of free water. Demeclocycline or lithium chloride helps treat chronic SIADH by impeding the renal response to ADH.

Evaluation

Base your evaluation on the expected outcomes listed on the nursing care plan. To determine if the patient's improved, ask yourself the following questions:
• Can the patient maintain a balanced fluid intake and output?
• Does his urine specific gravity fall within the normal range?
• Can he maintain normal weight?
• Has his mental status changed?

The answers to these questions will help you evaluate your patient's status and the effectiveness of his care. Keep in mind that these questions stem from the sample care plan above. Your questions may differ.

Pituitary Disorders

Self-Test

1. Anterior pituitary hormones include all of the following except:
a. prolactin   **b.** adrenocorticotropic hormone   **c.** vasopressin
d. luteinizing hormone

2. Which of the following visual changes may stem from a pituitary tumor?
a. nasal field loss in both eyes   **b.** temporal field loss in both eyes   **c.** nasal field loss in the right eye only   **d.** temporal field loss in the right eye only

3. If your patient's recovering from transsphenoidal hypophysectomy, be sure to assess him for:
a. pituitary apoplexy   **b.** diabetes insipidus   **c.** SIADH
d. empty-sella syndrome

4. Causes of secondary (acquired) renal diabetes insipidus include all of the following except:
a. increased sodium intake   **b.** protein deficiency
c. hypercalcemia   **d.** renal disease

5. If your patient has SIADH, expect his serum sodium level to:
a. remain the same   **b.** increase   **c.** decrease   **d.** increase initially, then decrease rapidly

6. Acromegaly signs and symptoms include all of the following except:
a. enlarged jaw and tongue   **b.** enlarged hands   **c.** excessive sweating   **d.** extreme height

7. For a child with growth hormone deficiency, the doctor will probably order:
a. somatrem   **b.** human growth hormone   **c.** glucocorticoids
d. mineralocorticoids

8. ADH has all of the following effects except:
a. promoting smooth muscle contraction   **b.** promoting vasoconstriction   **c.** helping dilute urine   **d.** acting as an antidiuretic

Answers (page number shows where answer appears in text)
1. **c** (page 19)   2. **b** (page 27)   3. **b** (page 36)   4. **a** (page 39)
5. **c** (page 43)   6. **d** (page 32)   7. **a** (page 35)   8. **b** (page 38)

Thyroid Disorders: Hyperthyroidism, Hypothyroidism, and Other Problems

Sande Jones, who wrote this chapter, is Inservice Education Coordinator, Department of Nursing Education, Mount Sinai Medical Center, Miami. She received her BSN from Southeastern Massachusetts University, North Dartmouth, and her MS in Adult Education from Florida International University, Miami. She is certified in Medical/Surgical Nursing by the American Nurses' Association.

Because thyroid hormones affect nearly all body tissues, disorders resulting from excessive or deficient thyroid hormone secretion can cause profound physiologic changes. Before reading about these disorders, first review thyroid gland anatomy (see *Thyroid gland structure*). To effectively assess and care for the patient with a known or suspected thyroid disorder, you'll also need to understand the three hormones produced by the thyroid gland: thyroxine (T_4), triiodothyronine (T_3)—collectively known as thyroid hormone—and calcitonin. (The thyroid gland alone produces T_4. Although it also produces T_3, other body tissues can also make this hormone by deiodinating T_4.)

Because iodine's the main component of thyroid hormone, the body must contain sufficient iodine for hormonal biosynthesis. The minimum daily iodine requirement's about 80 mcg, but many Americans get up to 500 mcg. Major iodine sources include seafood, water, bread, and iodized salt. With the increasing use of iodophors as sterilizing agents, even more iodine has entered the food chain.

Thyroid hormone production and release follow this sequence of events:
- iodide trapping
- iodide oxidation to iodine
- iodine organification into monoiodotyrosine
- iodinated precursor coupling
- hormone storage
- hormone release.

Trapping. After ingested iodine breaks down into iodide, the body absorbs iodide—mainly from the small intestine. Confined largely to extracellular fluid, iodide moves through the bloodstream. The kidneys remove most of it, excreting it in the urine. A minute amount enters the salivary glands, stomach, sweat glands, and breast milk. Thyroid tissue traps about a fourth of the iodide and actively moves it into thyroidal follicle cells. Various terms, including iodide trap, iodide pump, and iodide transport, describe the thyroid's iodide extraction from the blood.

Oxidation. Hydrogen peroxide and the membrane-associated enzyme peroxidase oxidize iodide, forming iodine.

Organification. This term describes the formation of the thyroid hormone precursors monoiodotyrosine (MIT) and diiodotyrosine (DIT) from the union of iodine and thyroglobulin (a colloid within follicle cells that contains 140 tyrosine molecules).

Coupling. MIT and DIT couple in the following ways to make thyroid hormone:
- Two DIT molecules form T_4
- One DIT molecule and one MIT molecule yield T_3 or reverse T_3 (rT_3).

When hormone synthesis ends, each thyroglobulin molecule may contain from five to six T_4 molecules and one T_3 molecule.

Storage. The thyroid gland—unique among endocrine glands—can store large hormone quantities for months in its follicle cells. This

Continued on page 50

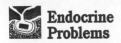
Thyroid Disorders

Thyroid gland structure

The thyroid gland—a butterfly-shaped structure weighing from 15 to 20 g—lies just below the larynx, in front and on either side of the trachea. The isthmus bridges the thyroid's left and right lobes across the trachea, just below the cricoid cartilage. The parathyroid glands lie on the posterior thyroid lobe surfaces.

Between the lobes, the recurrent laryngeal nerves run in the cleft separating the trachea and esophagus. The pyramidal lobe, a narrow thyroid tissue projection jutting upward from the isthmus, represents the embryonic thyroglossal tract.

Highly vascular, the thyroid gland receives blood from four major arteries arising from the external carotid and subclavian arteries. Many people have a fifth artery, arising from the aortic arch and entering the thyroid's midportion. Neurogenic stimuli regulate blood flow.

The thyroid receives nerve impulses from three sources:
• cervical ganglia (adrenergic innervation)
• vagus nerve (cholinergic innervation)
• adrenergic nerve fibers.

The thyroid contains follicular and parafollicular cells. Filled with a secretory substance called colloid and lined with an epithelium, follicle cells synthesize thyroxine (T_4) and triiodothyronine (T_3), collectively called thyroid hormone. Epithelial cells initiate thyroid hormone synthesis and trigger their release into the bloodstream. Thyroid hormone synthesis and storage take place in thyroglobulin, a colloid within follicle cells.

Parafollicular cells, also called C cells, lie in the follicles' basal portion. These cells secrete a third thyroid hormone—calcitonin, also known as thyrocalcitonin. Calcitonin rapidly reduces serum calcium levels.

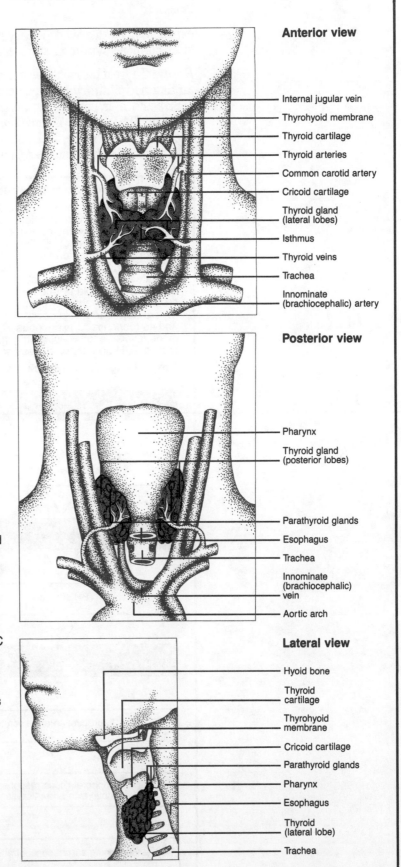

Anterior view

- Internal jugular vein
- Thyrohoid membrane
- Thyroid cartilage
- Thyroid arteries
- Common carotid artery
- Cricoid cartilage
- Thyroid gland (lateral lobes)
- Isthmus
- Thyroid veins
- Trachea
- Innominate (brachiocephalic) artery

Posterior view

- Pharynx
- Thyroid gland (posterior lobes)
- Parathyroid glands
- Esophagus
- Trachea
- Innominate (brachiocephalic) vein
- Aortic arch

Lateral view

- Hyoid bone
- Thyroid cartilage
- Thyrohyoid membrane
- Cricoid cartilage
- Parathyroid glands
- Pharynx
- Esophagus
- Thyroid (lateral lobe)
- Trachea

Thyroid Disorders

Continued

explains why a thyroid deficiency may not appear for several months after hormone synthesis stops completely.

Release. Thyroid hormone release depends on two other hormones—an anterior pituitary hormone called thyroid-stimulating hormone (TSH) and a hypothalamic hormone called thyrotropin-releasing hormone (TRH). (See *Thyroid hormone regulation.*) When the body needs thyroid hormone, TRH signals TSH, which, in turn, stimulates the thyroid gland. Stimulated thyroid cells send out pseudopod-like

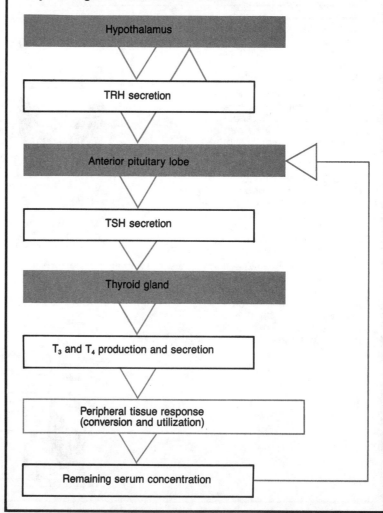

Thyroid hormone regulation

The hypothalamic-pituitary-thyroid axis and an autoregulatory thyroid gland mechanism regulate thyroid function. Hypothalamic neurons synthesize thyrotropin-releasing hormone (TRH), which then travels to anterior pituitary cells containing TRH-binding receptors. TRH secretion, in turn, triggers thyroid-stimulating hormone (TSH) in the anterior pituitary gland. Although TSH regulates most thyroid metabolism, it functions mainly to produce and secrete thyroid hormones. These hormones inhibit TSH secretion from the anterior pituitary gland. Minute changes in serum thyroid hormone levels cause reciprocal changes in TSH secretion and its response to exogenous TRH. When serum thyroid hormone levels become sufficiently high, the pituitary gland stops secreting TSH and becomes less sensitive to stimulation by TRH.

Thyroid negative feedback mechanism

Hypothalamus

TRH secretion

Anterior pituitary lobe

TSH secretion

Thyroid gland

T_3 and T_4 production and secretion

Peripheral tissue response
(conversion and utilization)

Remaining serum concentration

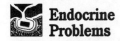
Thyroid Disorders

extensions to form pinocytotic vesicles around thyroglobulin. Fusing with lysosomes, the vesicles form digestive sacs. Inside these sacs, enzymes break down thyroglobulin, releasing T_4 and T_3; these substances then diffuse through the thyroid cell's base into the surrounding capillaries.

In the blood, T_4 and T_3 combine with several plasma proteins, including thyroxine-binding globulin (TBG), thyroxine-binding prealbumin (TBPA), and albumin. Only a small portion circulates freely—a quantity known as the free fraction. About every 6 days, half the protein-bound T_4 becomes available to tissue cells. Because T_3 has a lower binding affinity, half becomes free about every 1.3 days.

Several factors can inhibit thyroid hormone production and release. Thyroid hormone antagonists, such as propylthiouracil (PTU) and methimazole, can block the peroxidase enzyme system. Excessive iodine and lithium carbonate doses can inhibit thyroid hormone release.

We've already mentioned that thyroid hormone acts on most body tissues, generally stimulating them. Specifically, thyroid hormone has the following effects:

• *Metabolism.* Thyroid hormone increases the metabolic rate of most body tissues, accelerates food utilization for energy, speeds protein synthesis and catabolism, excites mental processes, and increases other endocrine gland functions.

• *Growth.* In children, thyroid hormone accelerates growth.

• *Carbohydrate metabolism.* Thyroid hormone stimulates most aspects of carbohydrate metabolism, including cellular glucose uptake, glycolysis, gluconeogenesis, gastrointestinal (GI) carbohydrate absorption, and insulin secretion.

• *Fat metabolism.* Thyroid hormone enhances fat metabolism, including lipid mobilization from fat tissues and free fatty acid oxidation.

• *Body weight.* In adults, thyroid hormone production usually relates inversely to body weight; for example, increased hormone production typically decreases weight. (However, because thyroid hormone stimulates the appetite, some hyperthyroid patients eat more and consequently *don't* lose weight.)

• *Cardiovascular function.* By accelerating metabolism, thyroid hormone causes vasodilation in most body tissues. As a result, blood flow increases, particularly to the skin, which requires blood for cooling. Increased blood flow also means increased cardiac output and heart rate, with arterial pressure rising as a result. However, if peripheral vessels dilate enough to accommodate the increased blood flow, arterial pressure may not rise. Pulse pressure, on the other hand, remains increased, so that systolic pressure may rise 10 to 20 mm Hg while diastolic pressure drops by the same amount.

• *Respiration.* The increased metabolic rate intensifies oxygen use and carbon dioxide formation, forcing respiratory rate and depth to rise.

• *GI function.* Thyroid hormone increases appetite, food absorption, digestive juice secretion, and GI tract motility (possibly leading to diarrhea).

• *Central nervous system function.* Thyroid hormone speeds mental processes and increases activity in spinal cord areas that control muscle tone.

Continued on page 52

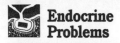
Thyroid Disorders

Reviewing thyroid hormones

Hormone	Releasing/inhibiting stimulus	Primary target site	Primary effects
Thyroxine (T_4) and triiodothyronine (T_3) (collectively called thyroid hormone)	Thyroid-stimulating hormone (TSH) from the anterior pituitary	Most body tissues	• Accelerate the body's metabolic rate and oxygen consumption
Calcitonin (thyrocalcitonin)	Serum ionized calcium level	Bone	• Modifies calcium metabolism

Continued

Synthesis of the third thyroid hormone, calcitonin, occurs in the parathyroid glands as well as in the thyroid gland. Calcitonin causes serum calcium effects opposing those of parathyroid hormone (PTH). Working rapidly, calcitonin can decrease the serum calcium level within minutes in three ways. First, it immediately decreases osteoclastic activity. About an hour later, it increases osteoblastic activity. Finally, it prevents precursor cells from forming new osteoclasts; this results in decreased osteoblastic activity.

Unlike PTH, which sets the long-term serum calcium level, calcitonin regulates short-term calcium ion concentration. Its effects last a few days at most.

Assessment

The patient's history and physical examination can provide valuable clues to a thyroid disorder.

History. Determine the patient's chief complaint by asking him why he's seeking medical attention. His answer could provide the first clue to thyroid dysfunction, even if it seems unrelated. Your next questions will depend on the chief complaint or on the patient's signs and symptoms. You might want to ask questions such as the following:
• Do you have trouble swallowing? Do you feel a lump, choking sensation, or pressure in your throat? (This could mean thyroid goiter or Hashimoto's disease [chronic autoimmune thyroiditis].)
• Have you noticed any skin changes? (Hyperthyroidism classically causes diaphoresis and facial flushing.)
• Has your tolerance to heat or cold changed? (Heat intolerance may indicate hyperthyroidism; cold intolerance, hypothyroidism.)
• Has your weight changed? (Hypothyroidism may cause a moderate weight gain; hyperthyroidism, a weight loss.)
• Have you felt any palpitations or "skipped" heartbeats? (Palpitations, tachycardia, and hypertension may result from hyperthyroidism.)

To obtain the patient's past medical and social histories, ask these questions:
• Do you use any medications—prescription or over-the-counter? (Some medications may cause or mask signs and symptoms of a thyroid disorder.)
• Have you ever been hospitalized or undergone medical treatment? Have you had radiation therapy or neck surgery? (Upper-body and neck surgery can cause thyroid disease or dysfunction.)
• Have you ever suffered head trauma? (A basal skull fracture may

Thyroid Disorders

Hyperthyroidism and hypothyroidism: Comparing assessment findings

Parameter	Hyperthyroidism	Hypothyroidism
Appearance	Exophthalmos, lid lag, impaired blinking	Swollen lips, thickened nose, impaired growth (in a child)
Basal metabolic rate	Increased	Decreased
Behavior	Restlessness, irritability, anxiety, hyperactivity, sleeplessness	Physical and mental sluggishness, somnolence, mental retardation (in an infant)
Cardiovascular system	Increased cardiac output, tachycardia, palpitations	Decreased cardiac output, bradycardia
Catecholamine sensitivity	Heightened	Reduced
Gastrointestinal system	Increased appetite, diarrhea	Decreased appetite, constipation
Integumentary system	Increased perspiration; thin, silky hair	Decreased perspiration; coarse, dry hair
Musculoskeletal system	Increased muscle tone and reflexes, tremors, twitching	Decreased muscle tone and reflexes
Respiratory system	Dyspnea	Hypoventilation
Serum cholesterol levels	Decreased	Increased
Temperature tolerance	Heat intolerance	Cold intolerance
Weight	Loss	Gain

lead to midbrain injury resulting in pituitary and hypothalamic dysfunction and subsequent TRH abnormality.)
• Do you drink alcohol or use recreational drugs? (Alcohol or drug intoxication or withdrawal can produce signs and symptoms that mimic a thyroid disorder.)
• As a child, was your growth accelerated or delayed? (Either pattern may indicate pituitary dysfunction.)
• Do you have an unusual appetite? (Thyroid hormones stimulate the appetite; a hyperthyroid patient may report a modest weight loss despite a hearty appetite. A hypothyroid patient may report a weight gain and may suffer anorexia, constipation, gaseous distention, fecal impaction, and achlorhydria.)
• Where do you live and work? (An iodine deficiency in local food and water may cause thyroid enlargement.)

With a woman, ask about her menstrual periods. Menorrhagia before menopause may indicate hypothyroidism; decreased menstrual flow may mean hyperthyroidism. Also find out if the patient has a family history of thyroid problems. Studies suggest a hereditary basis for Graves' disease and goiter.

Physical examination. Begin with inspection. Your patient's facial features may suggest thyroid dysfunction. Paleness, puffiness, and absent expression at rest suggest hypothyroidism. A frightened or anxious expression may indicate hyperthyroidism. Observe him as

Continued on page 54

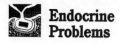
Thyroid Disorders

Continued

he talks. An enlarged tongue, deliberate speech, difficulty articulating, and a low-pitched, slow, husky voice all suggest hypothyroidism.

Next, check your patient's hair. Dry, brittle, and sparse hair may mean hypothyroidism. Fine, soft, silky hair characterizes hyperthyroidism. Hair that won't curl or hold a permanent may mean either hypothyroidism or hyperthyroidism.

Ask your patient about visual problems and look at his eyes. Exophthalmos (eyeball protrusion with obvious eyelid retraction) and eye prominence with diplopia both suggest Graves' disease. Eyelid swelling occurs commonly with both hypothyroidism and hyperthyroidism. Ask the patient to look down without moving his head. If you notice lid lag—failure of the upper eyelid to keep pace with the moving eyeball—suspect hyperthyroidism.

Observe your patient's neck for thyroid enlargement. Look at his hands and feet. Thickened, brittle nails and broadened hands and feet may indicate hypothyroidism. Elbow redness and Plummer's nails—separation of the nail edges from the nail bed—suggest hyperthyroidism.

Ask your patient if he's had any muscle aches. Then watch him as he gets out of a chair. Hyperthyroidism usually causes proximal muscle weakness and may lead to hyperactive reflexes. Ask the patient to extend his leg while seated in a chair. With hyperthyroidism, he may have trouble keeping his leg horizontal for more than 30 seconds (a normal person can sustain this position for about 2 minutes). To check for muscle tremor, have your patient spread his fingers in the air, palms down. Then place a piece of paper over his fingers. Paper movement indicates tremors—a possible sign of hyperthyroidism.

Next, perform palpation—the thyroid's the only endocrine gland you can feel. When palpating the thyroid, feel for a goiter—a glandular enlargement that may be diffuse or nodular. An enlarged thyroid may feel finely lobulated, like a well-defined organ. Determine the gland's consistency. A firm, hard enlargement may mean thyroiditis, goiter, or cancer. With any enlargement, check for asymmetry (which may mean cancerous goiter). Does the enlargement feel multinodular, or does it seem like a single lump? Nodules feel like knots, protuberances, or swellings; a solitary firm, fixed nodule may be a tumor. Report any lump beyond the thyroid's normal position; it may be a thyroglossal cyst. With an enlarged gland, check for tracheal displacement. Perform Kocher's test for tracheal compression by having the patient take a deep breath as you apply slight pressure to the thyroid's lateral lobes. Stridor on deep inspiration signals compression (see *Examining the thyroid gland* for more on palpation.)

Auscultation helps detect any bruits from an enlarged thyroid. A sign of turbulence from increased blood flow, a bruit indicates hyperthyroidism. Place the stethoscope's diaphragm over one of the thyroid's lateral lobes and listen for a soft, low, rushing sound. To rule out venous hum, gently occlude the patient's jugular vein. This will make any hum disappear. (*Note:* You'll skip percussion when examining the thyroid gland.)

Thyroid Disorders

Examining the thyroid gland

First inspect the patient's neck, identifying the thyroid gland, cricoid cartilage, and trachea. Note tracheal and thyroid contour and symmetry. Then, inspect and palpate the trachea for deviations. Observe the patient's neck as he extends it slightly. Offer him some water and watch while he swallows (this action raises the trachea, larynx, and thyroid). The trachea should be in midline position. Note any unusual thyroid bulging behind the sternocleidomastoid muscles.

Next, ask the patient to lower his chin slightly to relax the neck muscles and make examination easier. Standing in front of the patient, use the pads of your middle and index fingers to locate the cricoid cartilage. Ask him to swallow, then feel for the thyroid isthmus, located slightly below the cartilage.

Have the patient flex his head slightly forward and to the right. To palpate the thyroid's right lobe, place your right thumb on the lower thyroid cartilage, then grasp the sternocleidomastoid muscle with your left index and middle fingers. Use your left thumb to palpate the lobe by feeling in front of the muscle as the patient swallows.

To palpate the left lobe, switch hand positions and repeat the procedure.

You can also palpate your patient's thyroid from a posterior position. Standing behind the patient, rest your thumbs on the nape of his neck. Use the index and middle fingers of both hands to feel for the thyroid isthmus and the anterior lobe surfaces. With the patient's neck flexed forward and to the right, displace the thyroid cartilage to the right using your left hand. Use your right hand to palpate as the patient swallows. Your thumb should be placed deep behind the sternocleidomastoid muscle and your index and middle fingers in front.

In another, less common approach, you can stand at the patient's side, placing one hand behind and one hand in front of his neck. This position allows both inspection and palpation. To palpate both lobes, move from one side of the patient to the other, or turn your thumb down while palpating so that you can inspect the far lobe.

Note: The patient's physique and the thyroid gland's size will affect your ability to inspect and palpate.

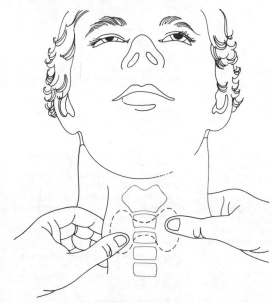

Left hand palpates; right hand displaces (anterior approach).

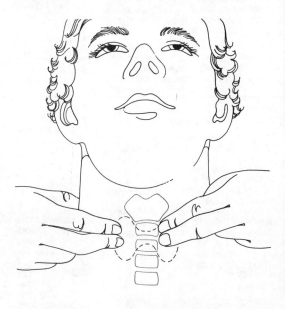

Right hand palpates; left hand displaces (posterior approach).

Diagnostic tests. Because no single test can determine thyroid status, expect the doctor to order various studies. Keeping in mind the patient's signs and symptoms, the doctor will interpret each test result in light of other findings.

The *thyroid panel* usually consists of the free T_3 and free T_4 tests and the T_3 and T_4 radioimmunoassays. To confirm or rule out hyperthyroidism, the doctor considers results of the total T_4, free T_4 index, and both T_3 tests. Along with the TSH assay, the total T_4 test and free T_4 index help diagnose hypothyroidism. If the T_3 and T_4 tests yield borderline results, the radioactive iodine uptake (RAIU) test and TSH assay may prove useful. The TSH and TRH

Continued on page 57

Thyroid Disorders

Selected laboratory tests

Serum triiodothyronine (T_3, T_3-RIA)
Determines total T_3 serum concentration. Preferred for diagnosing T_3 toxicosis (hyperthyroidism characterized by elevated T_3 and normal T_4 levels)

Implications of abnormal results:
Above-normal value suggests hyperthyroidism, T_3 toxicosis, acute thyroiditis, or idiopathic thyroxine-binding globulin (TBG) elevation. Below-normal value suggests hypothyroidism, starvation, idiopathic TBG depression, or acute illness.

Nursing considerations:
• Pregnancy and use of drugs such as T_3, estrogens, and antiovulatory preparations may increase values.
• Use of drugs such as anabolic steroids, androgens, phenytoin, T_4, and salicylates (in large doses) may decrease values.

Serum thyroxine (T_4, T_4-RIA)
Determines total circulating T_4 level by assessing ability of stable T_4 to displace radioactive T_4 from specific anti-T_4 antibody. Helps monitor potassium iodide therapy

Implications of abnormal results:
Above-normal value may indicate hyperthyroidism, acute thyroiditis, early-stage hepatitis, or idiopathic TBG elevation. Below-normal value may indicate hypothyroidism, chronic thyroiditis, nephrosis, or idiopathic TBG depression.

Nursing considerations:
• Administration of radioactive iodine tracer within 48 hours before test may alter test results.
• Use of drugs such as estrogens, antiovulants, and levothyroxine may increase values.
• Use of drugs such as androgens, anabolic steroids, salicylates, T_3, sulfonamides, phenytoin, and propranolol may decrease values.

Total T_4 (T_4 assay)
Directly measures total serum thyroxine concentration

Implications of abnormal results:
Above-normal value may indicate hyperthyroidism, acute or subacute thyroiditis, or early-stage hepatitis. Below-normal value may indicate cretinism, myxedema, or hypothyroidism.

Nursing considerations:
• Thyroid hormone therapy must be discontinued 1 month before test to ensure accurate results.
• Use of estrogens and anticonvulsant drugs may increase values.

Free T_4
Measures free (unbound) circulatory T_4 level; helps determine thyroid function, evaluate thyroid hormone replacement therapy, and rule out hypothyroidism and hyperthyroidism

Implications of abnormal results:
Above-normal value suggests

Graves' disease. Below-normal value suggests primary, secondary, or tertiary hypothyroidism or T_3 toxicosis.

Nursing considerations:
• Use of heparin causes false elevation.
• Test reliably evaluates thyroid status in pregnant patients with abnormal TBG values and in those taking estrogens, phenytoin, or salicylates.

Free T_4 index
Corrects estimated total T_4 level from TBG value (by multiplying T_4 value by T_3 uptake ratio). Assesses patients with known or suspected abnormal TBG level

Implications of abnormal results:
Above-normal value suggests hyperthyroidism. Below-normal value suggests hypothyroidism.

Nursing considerations:
• Test gives most accurate evaluation of thyroid status in patients taking estrogens, androgens, phenytoin, or salicylates.

Free T_3
Measures freely circulating T_3 fraction; helps rule out T_3 toxicosis, hypothyroidism, and hyperthyroidism; and helps monitor and evaluate thyroid hormone replacement therapy

Implications of abnormal results:
Above-normal value suggests hyperthyroidism or T_3 toxicosis. Below-normal value suggests hypothyroidism.

Nursing considerations:
• Inform laboratory personnel if patient has recently undergone test involving administration of radioactive material.

T_3 uptake ratio (T_3 resin uptake; serum T_4 binding capacity)
Indirectly measures unsaturated serum TBG level. A known amount of radioactive T_3 (which exceeds the capacity of TBG to bind to it) and a resin are added to a serum sample. Helps diagnose hyperthyroidism and hypothyroidism

Implications of abnormal results:
Above-normal value suggests hyperthyroidism, nephrosis, severe liver disease, metastatic cancer, or pulmonary insufficiency. Below-normal value suggests hypothyroidism or hyperestrogenic condition.

Nursing considerations:
• Use of such drugs as dicumarol, heparin, androgens, anabolic steroids, phenytoin, diphenylhydantoin, phenylbutazone, levothyroxine, thyroid USP, or salicylates (in large doses) may cause above-normal values.
• Pregnancy, menstruation, and use of such drugs as estrogens, oral contraceptives, thionamides, thiazide diuretics, chlordiazepoxide (Librium), and sulfonylureas may cause below-normal values.

Thyroglobulin (Tg)
Helps diagnose thyroid cancer and hyperthyroidism and monitors status of patients with thyroid cancer

Implications of abnormal results:
Above-normal value may indicate untreated or metastatic thyroid cancer, hyperthyroidism, subacute thyroiditis, or benign adenoma.

Nursing considerations:
• All samples must undergo screening for endogenous thyroglobulin antibodies, which invalidate test results.

Thyroxine-binding globulin (TBG)
Helps determine congenital TBG excess or deficiency and confirms thyroxine-binding protein abnormalities. Simultaneous TBG and T_4 testing accurately assesses thyroid function.

Implications of abnormal results:
Above-normal value suggests hyperthyroidism, genetic or idiopathic hepatic liver disease, or acute intermittent porphyria. Below-normal value suggests nephrotic syndrome, marked hypoproteinemia, liver disease, uncompensated acidosis, or acromegaly.

Nursing considerations:
• Pregnancy and use of such drugs as estrogens, oral contraceptives, and perphenazine may cause above-normal values. Use of androgens, anabolic steroids, phenytoin, and prednisone may cause below-normal values.

Serum thyroid-stimulating hormone (TSH)
Helps diagnose primary hypothyroidism in patients with thyroid failure from intrinsic disease; helps differentiate primary from secondary hypothyroidism

Implications of abnormal values:
Above-normal value may indicate primary hypothyroidism. Below-normal value may indicate hyperthyroidism or secondary or tertiary hypothyroidism.

Nursing considerations:
• TSH injection and use of lithium or potassium iodide can cause above-normal values. Use of T_3, salicylates, corticosteroids, or heparin may cause below-normal values.

Thyroid stimulation test
Differentiates primary from secondary hypothyroidism

Implications of abnormal results:
Absent thyroid response to TSH stimulation suggests primary thyroid failure. Normal response suggests pituitary or hypothalamic disorder.

Nursing considerations:
• Blood sampling takes place at timed intervals before and after I.M. TSH injection.

Continued

Thyroid Disorders

Selected laboratory tests
Continued

Thyroid stimulation test
Continued
● Dietary iodine may antagonize TSH stimulation and cause below-normal TSH value. If ordered, restrict dietary iodine. Document any large iodine intake, such as from seafood, large vitamin doses, salt, or iodine-containing expectorants.
● Some persons form antibodies against TSH, which may interfere with future thyroid stimulation test or may cause an allergic reaction to future TSH injection.

Thyroid suppression test (T_3 [Cytomel] thyroid suppression test)
Detects hyperthyroidism

Implications of abnormal test results:
Continued T_3 secretion indicates hyperthyroidism.

Nursing considerations:
● Before test, patient receives standard T_3 (Cytomel) dose daily for one week.

Thyrotropin-releasing hormone (TRH) stimulation test
Assesses anterior pituitary gland responsiveness and differentiates among primary, secondary, and tertiary hypothyroidism

Implications of abnormal results:
No response or a slight increase may indicate hyperthyroidism. A value two or three times higher than normal suggests primary hypothyroidism. No response may indicate secondary hypothyroidism. A delayed increase may indicate tertiary hypothyroidism (multiple TRH injections may be needed to induce appropriate response).

Nursing considerations:
● Patient receives 500 mcg bolus of TRH, then undergoes intermittent blood sampling. Maximum response occurs 20 minutes after injection.

Thyroid antibodies (thyroid-stimulating immunoglobulins [TSI];

long-acting thyroid stimulator [LATS])
Helps assess Graves' disease and Hashimoto's disease

Implications of abnormal results:
Above-normal level indicates Graves' disease or Hashimoto's disease.

Nursing considerations:
● Some patients without disease may show thyroid antibody titers.

Serum calcitonin
Helps diagnose thyroid cancer

Implications of abnormal results:
Above-normal value suggests medullary thyroid cancer, C-cell hyperplasia, chronic renal failure, pernicious anemia, Zollinger-Ellison syndrome, or cancer of the lung, breast, or pancreas.

Nursing considerations:
● Patient must fast overnight but may continue to drink water.

Continued

stimulation tests and the TSH suppression test help assess homeostatic controls, thyroid reserves, and feedback mechanisms.

(When evaluating test results, keep in mind that most thyroid hormone binds to protein in the bloodstream. Only the minute portion that remains free determines the patient's thyroid status.)

Some patients with thyroid dysfunction, such as those with acute and subacute thyroiditis, may have normal serum T_4 and T_3 levels. If so, the doctor will probably order other diagnostic tests, such as a thyroid scan, ultrasound, or needle biopsy. (For more information on laboratory tests, see *Selected laboratory tests.*)

Thyroid scan (RAIU test). A thyroid scan uses radioactive iodine, administered as a capsule, a liquid, or an I.V. infusion. By measuring the thyroid's radioactive iodine uptake, the test evaluates thyroid size, position, and function and helps differentiate among masses in the neck, tongue base, and mediastinum. Thyroid cancer, Hashimoto's disease, and hypothyroidism appear as areas of decreased iodine uptake. Hyperthyroidism, Graves' disease, and autonomous nodules show as areas of increased uptake.

Be sure to explain the test's purpose and procedure to your patient. Tell him how he'll receive the iodine and that he'll need to lie on his back with his neck extended as much as possible during the scan. Reassure him that the test uses only a small amount of radioactive material and that he won't become radioactive. Emphasize that the test doesn't cause pain, but that it may be time-consuming.

Advise him to eliminate iodine from his diet for at least 1 week before the test (unless he's undergoing the test to evaluate thyroid response to drugs). A thyroid scan should precede any X-ray test using a thyroid-blocking contrast agent. Because a thyroid scan involves radioactivity, the doctor won't order it for a pregnant patient.

Continued on page 58

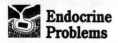
Thyroid Disorders

Continued

Thyroid ultrasound. Also called thyroid sonogram or echogram, this technique visualizes the thyroid by recording the reflection of ultrasonic waves directed into thyroid tissue. The doctor can then noninvasively assess the thyroid's size, differentiate a cyst from a solid tumor, and evaluate the depth and dimension of a thyroid goiter or nodule. Cystic, complex, or solid echo patterns indicate thyroid abnormalities.

To prepare your patient for ultrasound, explain that the procedure's painless and takes about 30 minutes. The patient will lie on a table with his neck hyperextended. The doctor may try to augment transducer contact by placing oil on the patient's skin or hanging a water-filled plastic bag over the patient's neck. Because it uses no radio-active materials, ultrasound can be used for a pregnant woman.

Hyperthyroidism

This disorder involves excessive thyroid hormone production resulting from thyroid disease, defective TSH or TRH, or thyroid hormone drug therapy. In some cases, it produces no apparent effects. When hyperthyroidism does cause signs and symptoms, it's known as thyrotoxicosis.

Causes of thyrotoxicosis fall into two categories:
• disorders associated with increased radioactive iodine uptake (for example, Graves' disease, toxic nodular goiter, and toxic adenoma)
• disorders associated with low radioactive iodine uptake (for example, subacute and silent thyroiditis).

Graves' disease, the most common cause of thyrotoxicosis, usually strikes women in their twenties and thirties, although a man or woman of any age may suffer from this condition. A multisystemic syndrome, Graves' disease affects the eyes, skin, and bones as well as the thyroid, commonly causing such problems as infiltrative ophthalmopathy, infiltrative dermopathy (myxedema), and acropachy (finger clubbing). Because most patients with Graves' disease have both hyperthyroidism and goiter, the condition's frequently called toxic diffuse goiter.

While researchers haven't identified the cause of Graves' disease, studies implicate abnormal T-lymphocyte function. A substance called thyroid-stimulating antibody (TSAb) apparently binds to TSH receptor sites on thyroid cells, preventing normal TSH binding. The autoantibody then activates the cells, causing uncontrolled hormone secretion.

Patients with Graves' disease typically suffer severe emotional stress just before symptoms arise. In some cases, symptoms follow a weight-reduction program involving severe dietary restriction, psychomotor stimulants (such as amphetamines), or thyroid hormone administration.

Assessment

Thyroid hormone's effects on other body regions usually provide the first clue to thyrotoxicosis. However, the patient may seek medical attention after noticing thyroid enlargement. Because thyroid hormone has stimulatory effects, expect signs and symptoms reflecting increased organ function (or an organ's inability to meet increased

Thyroid Disorders

Assessing hyperthyroidism

When assessing a patient for hyperthyroidism, stay alert for the following signs and symptoms:
- weight loss
- muscle wasting
- muscle weakness and tremor
- fatigue
- dyspnea
- breast enlargement
- palpitations
- increased appetite
- irritability and nervousness
- exophthalmos, lid lag
- profuse sweating
- heat intolerance.

Graves' disease—a form of hyperthyroidism—produces three characteristic signs:
- a uniformly enlarged thyroid gland (goiter)
- infiltrative ophthalmopathy
- infiltrative dermopathy.

(*Note:* All three signs may not appear in all patients.)

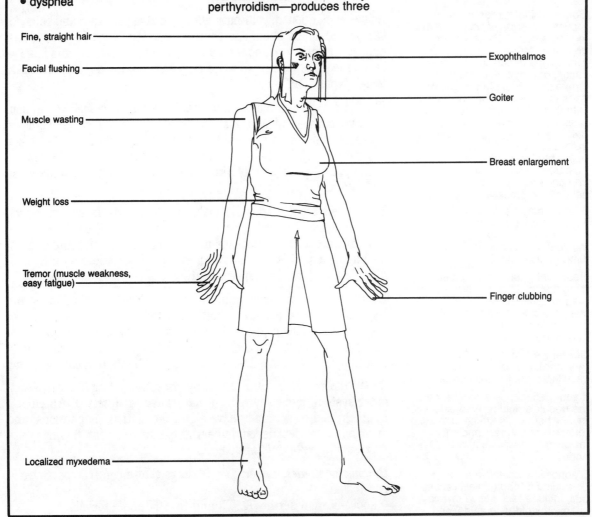

Fine, straight hair

Facial flushing

Muscle wasting

Weight loss

Tremor (muscle weakness, easy fatigue)

Localized myxedema

Exophthalmos

Goiter

Breast enlargement

Finger clubbing

demands). Specific findings depend on the patient's age and the rate of symptom onset. For example, an older patient with an abrupt symptom onset may have relatively severe signs and symptoms. In some patients, thyroid overstimulation causes especially marked effects on some organ systems (for example, the cardiovascular system suffers greater dysfunction in elderly patients).

If you suspect thyrotoxicosis, question your patient carefully about his family history—Graves' disease appears to be hereditary. Ask him about his eating habits; expect him to report an increased appetite but a slight weight loss. Find out how much iodine he consumes by asking if he eats a great deal of seafood or takes iodine-containing medications. Find out if he's had any breathing problems, such as dyspnea on exertion. Be sure to ask about temperature tolerance (thyrotoxicosis decreases heat tolerance).

Continued on page 60

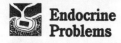
Thyroid Disorders

Goiter and nodules

Goiter. This term refers to a thyroid gland that's at least twice the normal size. A goiter may feel uniformly enlarged (diffuse goiter) or may contain small protuberant tissue masses (nodular goiter). A goiter may be nontoxic (euthyroid or hypothyroid) or toxic (hyperthyroid).

Goiters fall into three main groups. An *endemic goiter,* involving more than 10% of a given population group, usually results from iodine deficiency. In some cases, however, it stems from iodine excess and dietary goitrogens (substances that interfere with thyroid hormone production). A *sporadic goiter*—found in nonendemic goiter regions—results from a congenital thyroid hormone production defect, chemical agents, or iodine deficiency. A *compensatory goiter* follows partial thyroid removal.

A goiter may be discovered during a routine physical examination. Occasionally, a patient seeks medical attention after feeling a lump in his throat.

Treatment attempts to decrease thyroid size. Thyroid hormone preparations, such as levothyroxine, help block thyroid stimulation by suppressing thyroid-stimulating hormone secretion.

Solitary thyroid nodule. A solitary, hard, irregular nodule typically indicates thyroid cancer.

If your patient has a nodule, note the nodule's rigidity. Also determine whether it's attached to surrounding structures, and check for palpable regional lymph nodes.

Diagnostic studies, which help determine if the nodule's cancerous, include radioactive thyroid scans, thyroid ultrasound, and thyroid biopsy. Treatment of a solitary nodule may involve surgical removal or thyroid suppression with drugs such as levothyroxine.

Hyperthyroidism—*continued*

With a woman, ask about her menstrual pattern; be sure to note any decreased flow. (Also find out whether she's pregnant; the doctor will need this information when ordering diagnostic tests.)

Ask about eye problems, vision changes, and bowel habits. Hyperthyroidism stimulates GI tract motility, increasing bowel movement frequency and causing diarrhea.

As we've mentioned, your patient's general appearance and behavior can reveal much about his thyroid function. With thyrotoxicosis, expect the patient to appear nervous, irritable, restless, and fidgety; he'll probably speak rapidly. He may have a pained or apprehensive facial expression.

Check for exophthalmos, conjunctival edema, decreased visual acuity, and corneal ulcerations. Other characteristic facial signs of thyrotoxicosis include a wild or staring expression, lid lag when the patient rotates his eyes down, globe lag when he rotates his eyes up, and infrequent blinking. His forehead won't wrinkle when he looks up.

The patient's skin typically feels moist and warm and may look erythematous. Check his hair texture, which may be thin and fine. Note any alopecia. Inspect his nails (especially on the ring fingers) for Plummer's nails. His elbows may be red. A patient with Graves' disease may have hyperpigmentation and vitiligo.

Look for signs of tremor and muscle weakness in the hands and legs by having the patient hold them out. Be sure to check for thyroid enlargement and a thrill by carefully and gently palpating the gland. Expect it to feel firm but elastic. Auscultate for bruits, resulting from increased blood flow caused by thyroid enlargement.

Check the patient's vital signs. By overstimulating the cardiovascular system, hyperthyroidism may cause tachycardia. An elderly hyperthyroid patient may have atrial fibrillation, palpitations, and dyspnea. (For details on hyperthyroid assessment findings, see *Assessing hyperthyroidism,* page 59.)

Diagnostic studies. Laboratory findings that suggest hyperthyroidism include:
- above-normal serum T_3, T_4, and free T_3 and T_4 levels
- above-normal RAIU in Graves' disease and toxic nodular goiter; below-normal RAIU in thyroiditis
- above-normal radioactive T_3 uptake (RT_3U) level
- little or no TSH response to TRH stimulation
- below-normal serum TSH level
- positive thyroid-stimulating immunoglobulin test (in Graves' disease).

With thyrotoxicosis from cancer or multinodular goiter, a thyroid scan may aid diagnosis.

Planning
Before determining your nursing care plan, develop the nursing diagnosis by identifying your patient's problem or potential problem, then relating it to its cause. Possible nursing diagnoses for a patient with thyrotoxicosis include:
- injury, potential for (hypocalcemia); related to thyroidectomy

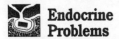

Thyroid Disorders

Thyroid storm

A life-threatening complication of hyperthyroidism, thyroid storm (also called thyroid crisis) has a high mortality. Signs and symptoms develop rapidly, triggered by such conditions as infection (especially pulmonary infection), sepsis, diabetes mellitus, trauma, severe stress, or abrupt thyroid medication withdrawal or overuse.

Signs and symptoms of thyroid storm include:
• fever (usually above 100° F. [37.8° C.])
• agitation and anxiety
• hot, flushed skin
• tachycardia
• systolic hypertension
• abdominal pain
• nausea and vomiting
• diarrhea
• anorexia
• dehydration.

As thyroid storm progresses, the patient may enter a stupor, then a coma. Hypotension and vascular collapse follow.

Thyroid storm can be difficult to diagnose because the precipitating condition may hinder its detection. Yet, the patient's survival hinges mainly on prompt clinical recognition.

Expect the doctor to order aggressive therapy, including the following interventions:
• maintaining airway patency and adequate breathing
• maintaining circulation with I.V. fluids, electrolytes (if needed), and continuous EKG monitoring
• administering thyroid hormone antagonists, such as propylthiouracil (PTU) and methimazole (Tapazole), to block thyroid hormone production and peripheral thyroid hormone effects
• administering iodine to inhibit thyroid hormone release
• administering a beta blocker, such as propranolol, to decrease thyroid hormone's accelerated cardiovascular and neuromuscular effects
• administering corticosteroids to block thyroid hormone secretion and extrathyroidal T_3 production
• correcting the precipitating illness or condition
• reducing fever with cooling blankets and nonsalicylate antipyretics. (*Important:* Don't give salicylates—they increase free thyroid hormone levels, thus exacerbating the patient's condition.)

• injury, potential for (eye injury); related to exophthalmos and lid lag
• nutrition, alteration in (less than body requirements); related to increased metabolism
• self-concept, disturbance in; related to physical appearance changes
• sleep pattern disturbances; related to increased metabolism
• anxiety; related to increased metabolism and nervous system irritation
• knowledge deficit; related to newly diagnosed disease.

The sample care plan below shows expected outcomes, nursing interventions, and discharge planning for one nursing diagnosis listed above. However, you'll want to individualize each care plan to fit the patient's needs.

Intervention

Treatment focuses on reducing elevated hormone levels and relieving hypermetabolic effects. Interventions may include:
• drugs, such as those that inhibit peripheral T_3 production and/or ameliorate excessive hormone effects
• radioiodine (^{131}I) therapy
• surgery (total or subtotal thyroidectomy).

Drugs. The thyroid hormone antagonists (thionamides) propylthiouracil (PTU) and methimazole (Tapazole) depress or inhibit thyroid hormone synthesis. PTU also inhibits production of T_3 from T_4 outside the thyroid. These drugs typically help treat children, adolescents, and pregnant women. The doctor may also order them to relieve thyrotoxicosis before thyroid surgery. Clinical improvement should appear after several weeks of therapy (as indicated by a serum T_4 reduction). After about a month, the doctor may reduce the dose by half or one third. Periodic laboratory tests determine

Continued on page 62

Sample nursing care plan: Hyperthyroidism

Nursing diagnosis	Expected outcomes
Injury, potential for (hypocalcemia); related to thyroidectomy	The patient will: • maintain a normal serum calcium level. • show negative Chvostek's and Trousseau's signs. • lack muscle twitching or finger numbness and tingling.

Nursing interventions	Discharge planning
• Observe patient for neuromuscular irritability. • Tell patient to immediately report any finger numbness or tingling. • Check for Chvostek's and Trousseau's signs every 2 hours. • Keep calcium gluconate available at bedside. • Monitor laboratory findings and notify doctor if serum calcium level decreases. • Discuss treatment and care plan with patient. • Discuss disease and its process with patient.	• Reinforce patient instructions. • Advise patient when to seek medical care, such as when signs and symptoms of hypocalcemia occur. • Arrange for follow-up medical care as necessary. • Discuss with patient any calcium replacement medication he must take at home, if indicated.

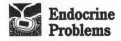
Thyroid Disorders

Subacute thyroiditis

This condition (also called giant cell, acute nonsuppurative, or granulomatous thyroiditis) ranks as the most common cause of thyroid pain and tenderness. Studies suggest it stems from a viral infection.

Subacute thyroiditis usually develops rapidly, typically accompanied by fever, chills, malaise, and muscle and joint pain. Upper respiratory infection commonly precedes the condition. Pain may radiate to the upper neck, ears, throat, or jaw. The thyroid gland enlarges—either diffusely or in a single lobe. On palpation, the gland may feel firm or even hard. About half the patients have clinical evidence of hyperthyroidism.

With mild subacute thyroiditis, the patient may recover without treatment. But most patients need anti-inflammatory drugs, such as salicylates, to relieve pain. Patients who don't respond to salicylates may get relief from prednisone. Besides relieving signs and symptoms, anti-inflammatory drugs probably inhibit thyroid hormone release, helping to reverse hyperthyroidism.

Most patients recover within a few weeks or months, although the condition may recur. A few suffer persistent neck pain and thyroid enlargement. Some require propranolol to relieve hyperthyroid symptoms.

Hyperthyroidism—*continued*

the need for further dose reductions until the patient reaches a maintenance dose.

Remind your patient to take his medication regularly—thionamides have a short half-life. Also tell him to watch for allergic reactions and agranulocytosis symptoms, such as fever, sore throat, and rash. If these symptoms occur, he should stop the medication and call his doctor immediately. Routine white blood cell counts help rule out neutropenia.

Once remission occurs, the doctor may stop drug therapy. However, the patient should have medical checkups every 2 to 3 months for the first year of remission, then annually.

Iodine and lithium carbonate therapy also inhibit thyroid hormone synthesis and release. Although iodine treatment's not used as the sole therapy for thyrotoxicosis, it may follow ^{131}I therapy or precede thyroidectomy. (Iodine may also help treat thyroid storm.) Lithium carbonate can be used alone, but its common adverse effects—depression, tremor, nausea, vomiting, and renal diabetes insipidus—limit its use. The doctor may order lithium for a patient who can't tolerate PTU or methimazole.

PTU, corticosteroids, propranolol, ipodate (Oragrafin), and iopanoic acid (Telepaque) help treat thyrotoxicosis by inhibiting T_4 conversion to T_3 outside the thyroid. A beta-adrenergic blocker, propranolol also helps control diaphoresis, palpitations, and anxiety.

[131]I therapy. This treatment, which works by partially destroying the thyroid, avoids the complications of surgery. Because benefits may not occur for weeks or even months, the doctor may order propranolol for symptomatic relief before and after ^{131}I therapy. A patient with severe symptoms may also need antithyroid medication until 2 to 3 days before ^{131}I therapy begins.

Although this treatment requires only a single dose, it almost always causes hypothyroidism (usually in the first few months after therapy). Because ^{131}I can cross the placenta and destroy the fetal thyroid gland, a pregnant woman should never undergo this treatment.

Surgery. Because they're simple, safe, and economical, antithyroid drugs and ^{131}I therapy have all but replaced subtotal thyroidectomy. However, the doctor may perform thyroidectomy in a child or adolescent who doesn't respond to other treatments, in a pregnant patient, or in one who refuses radioactive therapy. Patients with nodules, thyroiditis, cancer, or diffuse goiters that cause cosmetic or breathing problems also require surgery.

Because surgery can cause thyroid storm, expect your patient to receive antithyroid drugs preoperatively to maintain normal thyroid function. Iodine, such as Lugol's solution or saturated solution of potassium iodide (SSKI) helps firm the thyroid and, by reducing its vascularity, helps prevent postoperative hemorrhage. Give the iodine solution in milk or orange juice to make it more palatable. Be sure to watch for signs of iodine toxicity, such as buccal mucosal swelling, excess salivation, and skin reactions. Your patient may also receive propranolol preoperatively to decrease pulse rate and tremors.

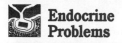
Thyroid Disorders

Thyroid cancer

Most thyroid cancers grow slowly and cause delayed symptoms. Typically, a solitary thyroid nodule's the first sign.

Thyroid cancers occur in four distinct histologic types. The most common, *papillary carcinoma,* usually strikes women under age 40. The tumor may remain localized for years before spreading to cervical lymph nodes. Eventually, this cancer may become aggressive and spread extensively.

Follicular carcinoma, the second most common type, also grows slowly. However, it's more likely to invade blood vessels and spread to bone and lung tissue. It less frequently spreads to local lymph nodes, but may adhere to the trachea, neck muscles, skin, and great vessels. Hoarseness and coughing occur when the tumor traps the recurrent laryngeal nerves.

Medullary carcinoma accounts for 5% to 10% of thyroid cancers. These tumors grow slowly, but spread to local lymph nodes. Death may result from distant metastases. Medullary cancer typically accompanies Sipple's syndrome or multiple endocrine neoplasia Type II or Type III. The parafollicular (C) cells that produce this tumor synthesize excess calcitonin and, less commonly, excess adrenocorticotropic hormone, prostaglandins, and serotonin.

Anaplastic carcinoma, an extremely aggressive tumor, grows rapidly, producing severe local symptoms. It spreads swiftly to lymph and blood vessels, sometimes causing death within 1 to 2 years.

Radiation-induced thyroid cancer. Radiation can cause thyroid cancer (most commonly, papillary carcinoma) up to 35 years after exposure. The radiation dose and the interval before cancer appearance seem unrelated. Radiation-induced thyroid cancer strikes adults and children equally.

Intervention. Treatment for thyroid cancer depends on the cancer type. Interventions include surgery, radioiodine (^{131}I) therapy, and thyroid hormone therapy.

Before surgery, teach the patient how to perform coughing and deep-breathing exercises and show him how to support his head and do range-of-motion neck exercises. Explain that he'll experience hoarseness and will have trouble talking for a few days after surgery from endotracheal tube placement and neck soreness. If your patient expresses concern about neck scarring, explain that the doctor will probably make the incision in a natural skin crease. Also suggest that the patient wear clothing that conceals the scar until it heals.

During surgery, the patient will lie on the operating table with his neck extended. The doctor will make a symmetrical low collar incision about ⅜″ to ¾″ (1 to 2 cm) above the clavicle and will create skin flaps to expose the area.

After establishing homeostasis around the wound, the doctor inserts a drain in the thyroid lobe bed, then brings the drain out through a small stab wound below the incision and closes the wound.

After surgery, assess your patient's vital signs, voice level, and neuromuscular function. Check his dressing carefully. Expect moderate drainage; lack of drainage may mean hematoma development. Also check behind the patient's neck (excessive bleeding may not appear on the front of the dressing).

Watch for respiratory distress, which may result from edema, bleeding, hematoma, tracheal compression, or laryngeal stridor from tetany or paralysis. Keep the patient in semi-Fowler's position and carefully support his neck to avoid suture-line tension. Administer analgesics, as ordered, to control incisional pain. Keep emergency supplies—oxygen, suctioning equipment, and a tracheostomy tray—at the patient's bedside; make sure calcium gluconate's readily available.

Monitor the patient for signs and symptoms of hypothyroidism. Usually transient, hypothyroidism resolves once thyroid hormone production returns to normal. Also stay alert for other complications, including the following:
• temporary sensation loss above the incision, from severed sensory nerves
• damage to one or both recurrent laryngeal nerves, resulting in hoarseness or total voice loss
• damage to the parathyroid glands or their blood supply, causing postoperative hypocalcemia and tetany (To avoid this problem, some surgeons resect, mince, and transplant the parathyroid glands into the sternocleidomastoid muscle.)
• superior thyroid artery damage, resulting in severe hemorrhage
• tracheal damage, resulting in aspiration of blood through the trachea or postoperative tracheocutaneous fistula formation.

Tell your patient to expect drain removal probably within 24 to 48 hours after surgery. The sterile dressing strips or staples closing the wound will probably remain in place for 10 days. The day after surgery, encourage him to get up and move around, as ordered; also start liquids and progress to a soft diet as soon as the patient can tolerate it. Unless he has complications, he can probably go home 2 to 6 days after surgery.

Continued on page 64

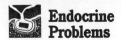
Thyroid Disorders

Hyperthyroidism—*continued*

Evaluation

Base your evaluation on the expected outcomes listed on your nursing care plan. To determine if the patient's improved, ask yourself the following questions:
- Does the patient's serum calcium level fall within a normal range?
- Does he have a positive Chvostek's or Trousseau's sign?
- Does he experience any muscle twitching or complain of numbness and tingling?
- Does he understand his treatment and care plan?

The answers to these questions will help you evaluate your patient's status and the effectiveness of his care. Keep in mind that these questions stem from the sample care plan on page 61. Your questions may differ.

Hypothyroidism

Inadequate peripheral-tissue thyroid hormone levels produce the signs and symptoms collectively known as hypothyroidism. The disease may be primary, secondary, or tertiary. Primary hypothyroidism results from thyroid tissue loss or atrophy; secondary hypothyroidism, from a pituitary defect that causes insufficient thyroid stimulation; tertiary hypothyroidism, from a hypothalamic defect causing insufficient thyroid stimulation. In rare instances, hypothyroidism may result from decreased peripheral-tissue sensitivity, resistance to thyroid hormones, or an exogenous cause (for example, iodine deficiency or use of drugs such as lithium).

Hypothyroidism takes three main forms: adult hypothyroidism, cretinism, and juvenile hypothyroidism. In this section, we'll focus on adult hypothyroidism. For information on other forms of hypothyroidism, see *Cretinism and juvenile hypothyroidism*.

Thyroid gland destruction—by disease or by treatment for thyrotoxicosis—most commonly causes adult hypothyroidism (also called myxedema or, when it causes thyroid atrophy, Gull's disease). Less common causes include inherited biosynthetic defects, iodine deficiency, and hormone synthesis inhibition by drugs or other chemicals.

A patient with adult hypothyroidism suffers various problems associated with low thyroid hormone levels, including arteriosclerosis (from elevated serum lipoprotein levels) and widespread deposition of interstitial glycosaminoglycan, which causes the characteristic mucinous edema (myxedema).

Assessment

A patient with hypothyroidism may complain of the following:
- changed sleeping habits (he may report sleeping up to 16 hours a day)
- lethargy, lack of ambition and concentration, and memory lapses
- headaches
- modest weight gain despite appetite loss
- cold intolerance
- dyspnea
- constipation, abdominal gas, or fecal impaction
- menorrhagia (in a woman)

Cretinism and juvenile hypothyroidism

Cretinism refers to profound hypothyroidism in infants. Because all developmental aspects depend on thyroid hormones, cretinism causes both physical and mental retardation. Left untreated, it leads to permanent brain damage. However, retardation can be prevented by early thyroid hormone replacement therapy.

Juvenile hypothyroidism begins during childhood—most commonly, from chronic autoimmune thyroiditis (Hashimoto's disease), drug therapy, or defective thyroid hormone synthesis. Affecting growth and sexual maturation, juvenile hypothyroidism usually produces signs and symptoms resembling those of adult hypothyroidism (myxedema).

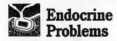
Thyroid Disorders

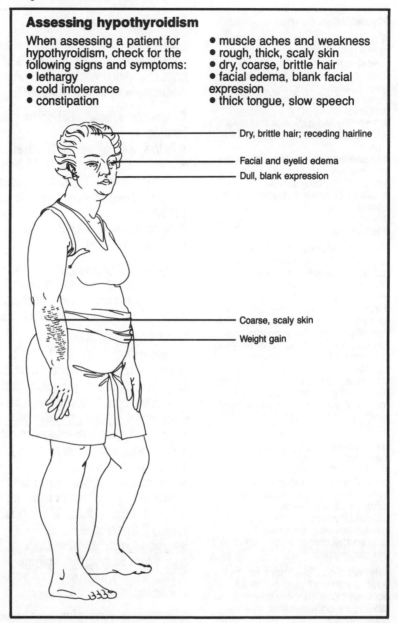

Assessing hypothyroidism

When assessing a patient for hypothyroidism, check for the following signs and symptoms:
- lethargy
- cold intolerance
- constipation
- muscle aches and weakness
- rough, thick, scaly skin
- dry, coarse, brittle hair
- facial edema, blank facial expression
- thick tongue, slow speech

Dry, brittle hair; receding hairline

Facial and eyelid edema

Dull, blank expression

Coarse, scaly skin

Weight gain

- muscle aches and weakness
- arm or leg paresthesia, delayed deep tendon reflex relaxation, and tingling hands (a sign of carpal tunnel syndrome, which results from medial nerve compression).

The patient may also have a history of anorexia (resulting from decreased metabolic activity) and a family history of thyroid dysfunction. Ask about his medication history; many drugs can cause hypothyroidism. Because hypothyroidism reduces red blood cell production, be sure to assess your patient for signs and symptoms of anemia.

When performing the physical examination, inspect the patient's face for lack of expression and puffiness (from mucopolysaccharide skin infiltration). His skin may feel cool and dry and may have an ivory or yellow tint (from carotene accumulation). The skin may also appear rough, thick, and scaly. Scalp hair may be dry, coarse, brittle, and lusterless. Eyebrows commonly become thin, disap-

Continued on page 66

Thyroid Disorders

Myxedema coma

A medical emergency, myxedema coma presumably involves progressive respiratory center depression, decreased cardiac output, and worsening cerebral hypoxia. Precipitating factors may include:
• thyroid medication withdrawal
• chronic untreated hypothyroidism
• acute illness, such as infection, in a patient with mild or undiagnosed hypothyroidism
• use of sedatives, narcotics, or anesthetics
• surgery
• exposure to cold.

These conditions lead to respiratory acidosis and carbon dioxide narcosis—a result of hypoventilation (common in hypothyroid patients, who have decreased respiratory drive or muscle dysfunction). And because long-term hypothyroidism may enlarge the tongue, myxedema coma may also result from a tongue-obstructed airway. Hyponatremia, decreased serum osmolarity, and abnormally concentrated urine may also alter mental status and produce coma in a hypothyroid patient.

Assessment. Expect signs and symptoms of hypothyroidism, such as bradycardia and hypotension. Respiratory depression and hypothermia (from reduced metabolism) may precede the coma. Laboratory test results, such as low serum total and free T_4 (serum thyroxine) levels, confirm the diagnosis.

Intervention. Treatment for myxedema coma should begin as soon as possible—usually before laboratory confirmation. Interventions include:
• maintaining airway patency with ventilatory support if necessary (respiratory failure commonly causes death)
• maintaining circulation via I.V. fluid replacement (with continuous EKG monitoring to assess cardiac status)
• monitoring arterial blood gases to detect metabolic acidosis
• passively warming the patient by wrapping him in blankets (*Important:* Don't use a warming blanket because it may increase peripheral vasodilation, causing shock.)
• monitoring body temperature with a low-reading thermometer
Continued

Hypothyroidism—*continued*

pearing at the ends. The patient's tongue may be enlarged, his speech slow and deliberate, and his voice hoarse and low-pitched from thickened vocal cords. (For details on hypothyroid assessment findings, see *Assessing hypothyroidism,* page 65.)

Diagnostic studies. Laboratory findings suggesting hypothyroidism include:
• below-normal serum T_4, free T_3, and free T_4 levels
• above-normal serum TSH level in primary hypothyroidism
• above-normal TRH stimulation response in primary hypothyroidism; poor or prolonged response in secondary or tertiary hypothyroidism
• below-normal RAIU
• below-normal RT_3U.

Other findings suggesting hypothyroidism include above-normal muscle enzyme levels (especially creatine phosphokinase); anemia (typically normochromic normocytic); and bradycardia, flattened or inverted T waves, heart block, and nonspecific ST segment changes on EKG.

Planning

Before determining your nursing care plan, develop the nursing diagnosis by identifying your patient's problem or potential problem, then relating it to its cause. Possible nursing diagnoses for a patient with hypothyroidism include:
• knowledge deficit; related to thyroid hormone replacement therapy
• nutrition, alteration in (less than body requirements); related to decreased metabolism
• self-concept, disturbance in; related to body changes
• skin integrity, impairment of; related to edema and dry skin
• bowel elimination, alteration in (constipation); related to decreased GI tract motility
• cardiac output, alteration in (decreased); related to decreased heart rate and stroke volume
• communication, impaired verbal; related to enlarged tongue and thickened vocal cords.

The sample care plan on the opposite page shows expected outcomes, nursing interventions, and discharge planning for one nursing diagnosis listed above. However, you'll want to tailor each care plan to meet your patient's needs.

Intervention

A hypothyroid patient requires lifelong thyroid hormone replacement therapy tailored to his specific needs. Synthetic thyroid hormones effectively relieve signs and symptoms and reverse the biochemical abnormalities caused by hypothyroidism. The doctor may order one of three synthetic preparations—most commonly, levothyroxine, also called T_4 (Synthroid, Levoid, Levothroid, Noroxine). The patient will probably begin levothyroxine treatment with a fairly low dose that the doctor increases every 1 to 3 weeks until achieving the desired response. An elderly patient or one with a known cardiac problem usually starts with a much smaller dose (carefully monitor such a patient for angina and cardiac dysrhythmias). A lactose-sensitive

Thyroid Disorders

Myxedema coma
Continued

- replacing thyroid hormone by administering large I.V. levothyroxine doses
- replacing fluids and other substances (such as glucose)
- administering corticosteroids, such as hydrocortisone
- treating any underlying illness (such as infection).

The patient's prognosis depends on the coma's duration and the promptness of treatment. Approximately 50% to 80% of patients die.

Sample nursing care plan: Hypothyroidism

Nursing diagnosis	Expected outcomes
Knowledge deficit; related to thyroid hormone replacement therapy	The patient will: • show he understands the action, dose, route of administration, and potential adverse effects of his thyroid medications. • show he understands why he needs to take his medication as prescribed. • maintain compliance with therapy.
Nursing interventions	**Discharge planning**
• Discuss with patient and his family the action, dose, route of administration, and potential adverse effects of his thyroid medication. • Discuss the disease and its signs and symptoms. • Discuss the importance of complying with therapy and ways to improve compliance, such as cuing techniques.	• Reinforce treatment and care plan. • Reinforce medication instructions. • Advise patient when to seek medical care. • Arrange for follow-up medical care, as indicated.

patient may show intolerance to Levothroid tablets, which contain lactose.

The doctor may choose liothyronine sodium (T_3 [Cytomel]), for a more rapid effect. The third synthetic hormone, liotrix (Euthroid), combines T_3 and T_4. The patient takes the drug orally, once a day. If he develops a headache while taking liotrix, he may need a dose reduction or a medication change.

Although doctors usually prescribe synthetic hormones because of their greater reliability, some patients may benefit from crude hormone preparations from cow or pig thyroids. Available extracts include desiccated thyroid USP (S-P-T, Thyrar, Thyro-Teric) and thyroglobulin (Proloid).

If your patient's taking any of these drugs, advise him to continue the medication even if he feels better. Make sure he can identify signs and symptoms of both hypothyroidism and hyperthyroidism to help monitor the medication's effectiveness. Encourage him to carry medical identification informing medical personnel of his hormone therapy. Also tell him to notify other health care workers about his hormone therapy; thyroid medications may potentiate or interact with various drugs.

Evaluation

Base your evaluation on the expected outcomes listed on the nursing care plan. To determine whether your patient's improved, ask yourself the following questions:
- Does the patient understand why he must take his thyroid medication regularly?
- Does he know the action, dose, route of administration, and potential adverse effects of his medication?
- Can he describe signs and symptoms of hypothyroidism and hyperthyroidism?
- Can he maintain his own medication therapy at home? If not, will a family member or friend help him?
- Does the patient know of other medications that may interact adversely with his thyroid medications?

Continued on page 68

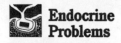
Thyroid Disorders

Hypothyroidism—*continued*

The answers to these questions will help you evaluate your patient's status and the effectiveness of his care. Keep in mind that these questions stem from the sample nursing care plan on page 67. Your questions may differ.

Self-Test

1. Hypothyroidism signs and symptoms include all of the following except:
a. exophthalmos   b. cold intolerance   c. constipation   d. weight gain despite appetite loss

2. Hyperthyroidism signs and symptoms include all of the following except:
a. lid lag   b. warm, moist, erythematous skin   c. Plummer's nails   d. lethargy

3. Of the following drugs, which is a thyroid hormone antagonist used to treat hyperthyroidism?
a. propranolol   b. levothyroxine   c. methimazole   d. liotrix

4. Postoperative nursing care for a patient who's had a thyroidectomy includes all of the following except:
a. keeping sodium bicarbonate at the bedside   b. checking behind the patient's neck for drainage   c. expecting moderate drainage on the patient's neck dressing   d. keeping the patient in semi-Fowler's position

5. Which of the following drugs probably won't be ordered for a hypothyroid patient?
a. Tapazole   b. Synthroid   c. Cytomel   d. Proloid

6. Be sure to ask your patient to swallow when assessing his thyroid gland, because swallowing makes the thyroid:
a. shift upward   b. shift downward   c. disappear   d. bulge

7. Signs and symptoms of thyroid storm include all of the following except:
a. fever (usually above 100° F. [37.8° C.])   b. dehydration   c. systolic hypertension   d. bradycardia

8. If your patient experiences thyroid storm, expect the doctor to order all of the following measures except:
a. inserting an I.V. line   b. administering a thyroid hormone antagonist   c. administering iodine   d. reducing fever by giving salicylates

9. Which of the following steps should you avoid when caring for a patient suffering myxedema coma?
a. replacing fluids   b. administering I.V. levothyroxine   c. administering corticosteroids   d. using a warming blanket to increase body temperature

Answers (page number shows where answer appears in text)
1. **a** (pages 64 to 65)   2. **d** (page 60)   3. **c** (page 61)   4. **a** (page 63)   5. **a** (pages 61; 66 to 67)   6. **a** (page 55)   7. **d** (page 61)   8. **d** (page 61)   9. **d** (page 66)

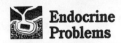
Parathyroid Disorders: Hyperparathyroidism, Hypoparathyroidism, and Other Problems

Jean Croce, who wrote this chapter, is a Nurse Practitioner who teaches critical care courses as an independent consultant. She received her BSN and MSN from the University of Tennessee, Knoxville. She has also earned her CCRN.

A parathyroid disorder may involve hyperfunction (hyperparathyroidism, which results in hypercalcemia) or hypofunction (hypoparathyroidism, which leads to hypocalcemia). To proceed correctly through effective assessment, planning, intervention, and evaluation of a patient with such a disorder, first expand your knowledge base by reviewing how the parathyroid glands control calcium and phosphate metabolism.

Continued on page 70

Parathyroid gland anatomy

The tiny parathyroid glands, which range from dark tan to yellow in adults, each weigh about 30 mg. Most people have four, but some have as many as six or as few as two. The glands usually occur in two pairs. The superior pair sit behind the middle and upper thirds of each thyroid lobe, next to the recurrent laryngeal nerve as it enters the larynx. The inferior pair lie behind the lower thyroid lobes, embedded in thyroid tissue, or within the thymus gland or the anterior superior mediastinum. If the usual locations contain fewer than four glands, ectopic glands may exist. The terminal interior thyroid artery branches supply the parathyroids with blood.

The parathyroids contain two cell types. *Chief cells,* the predominant type, synthesize and secrete parathyroid hormone (PTH, also called parathormone). *Oxyphil cells,* which appear after puberty and become more numerous with age, may be a degenerative chief cell form.

Besides PTH, the parathyroids produce some calcitonin (also called thyrocalcitonin), although this hormone's produced and secreted mainly by the thyroid gland.

With their small size and variable color and location, the parathyroids can be hard to identify; this sometimes results in their accidental removal during thyroid or other neck surgery. Loss of one or two glands usually doesn't affect function—one gland or even a partial gland can expand to supply enough hormones for calcium homeostasis. However, loss of three or four glands usually triggers temporary hypoparathyroidism.

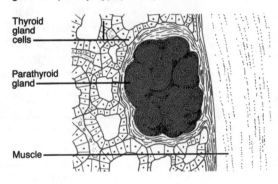

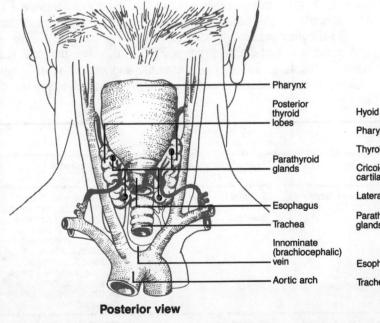

Posterior view

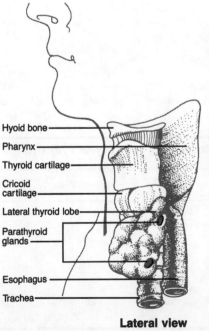

Lateral view

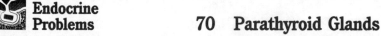

Parathyroid Disorders

Reviewing common terms

Absorption. Passage of substances into or across such tissues as the skin, intestines, and kidney tubules.

Bone mineralization. Bone formation through deposition of minerals, such as calcium and phosphate.

Bone resorption. Bone demineralization; migration of minerals from bone into blood, resulting from osteoclastic activity.

Renal excretion. Removal of substances from blood into the renal tubules for urinary excretion.

Renal reabsorption. Movement of substances from the renal tubules back into blood.

Continued

By regulating calcium and phosphate homeostasis, the parathyroid glands maintain appropriate serum levels. Regulation occurs mainly through the interaction of three substances—parathyroid hormone (PTH; also called parathormone), calcitonin, and vitamin D. These substances act at three target sites—the gastrointestinal (GI) tract, kidneys, and bone. PTH acts directly on the kidneys and bone; indirectly, through vitamin D, on the GI tract.

PTH activity. A polypeptide secreted by the parathyroid glands, PTH corrects serum calcium deficiency (hypocalcemia) by promoting calcium conservation by the kidneys, stimulating calcium release by bone, enhancing calcium absorption from the GI tract (in concert with vitamin D), and reducing serum phosphate levels.

A negative feedback mechanism controls PTH secretion: A reduced serum calcium level stimulates PTH release; an increased serum calcium level suppresses its release. Magnesium also affects PTH secretion by helping to mobilize calcium and by inhibiting PTH release when magnesium concentrations rise above normal or drop severely below normal. An increased serum phosphate level indirectly stimulates parathyroid activity: Renal tubular phosphate reabsorption triggers calcium secretion into the urine; the resulting serum calcium decrease then stimulates PTH secretion.

In the kidneys, PTH enhances tubular calcium reabsorption directly by increasing calcium reabsorption and phosphate excretion. Thus, the serum calcium level increases while the serum phosphate level decreases. Without reabsorption, urinary calcium excretion would eventually cause extensive bone decalcification. PTH also enhances urinary excretion of sodium, potassium, amino acids, and bicarbonate. Bicarbonate loss produces mild acidosis, which enhances bone resorption and increases calcium and phosphate release. PTH also stimulates the renal conversion of 25-hydroxycholecalciferol to 1,25-dihydroxycholecalciferol ($1,25[OH]_2D_3$; calcitriol). This active vitamin D metabolite permits PTH's full effect on bone. (Biologically inactive, dietary and ultraviolet-induced vitamin D must undergo two chemical alterations in the liver and kidneys to become active.)

Reviewing parathyroid hormones

Hormone	Releasing/inhibiting stimulus	Primary target site	Primary effects
Parathyroid hormone (PTH, parathormone)	Serum calcium concentration, vitamin D	Skeletal bone, kidney (renal tubules), and gastrointestinal tract	• Increases serum calcium level by decreasing renal calcium excretion, increasing GI tract calcium absorption, and increasing calcium migration from bone • Decreases serum phosphate (phosphorus) level by blocking renal tubular reabsorption
Calcitonin (thyrocalcitonin; mostly produced in thyroid gland)	Serum ionized calcium concentration	Skeletal bone	• Maintains serum calcium level mainly by inhibiting bone resorption by lowering serum calcium level (counterregulates PTH)

Parathyroid Disorders

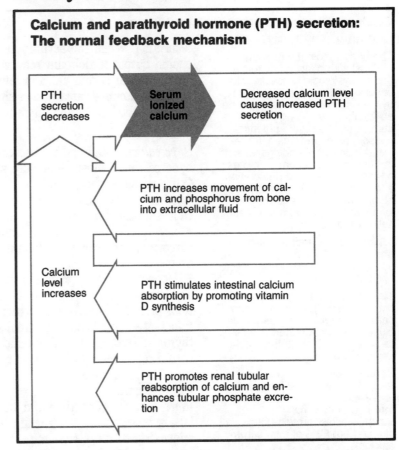

Calcium and parathyroid hormone (PTH) secretion: The normal feedback mechanism

PTH secretion decreases

Serum Ionized calcium

Decreased calcium level causes increased PTH secretion

PTH increases movement of calcium and phosphorus from bone into extracellular fluid

Calcium level increases

PTH stimulates intestinal calcium absorption by promoting vitamin D synthesis

PTH promotes renal tubular reabsorption of calcium and enhances tubular phosphate excretion

PTH also increases bone resorption through its direct action on bone and helps convert osteoblasts (bone-forming cells) to osteoclasts (cells involved in bone breakdown). By stimulating osteoclastic activity, PTH promotes bone breakdown and subsequent calcium release and serum calcium elevation. Normally, bone breakdown and buildup remain balanced to maintain constant bone mass. However, prolonged PTH elevation results in widespread bone resorption, causing bone erosion.

PTH apparently affects the GI tract indirectly, with calcitriol mediating its action by stimulating calcium absorption from the duodenum and upper jejunum (calcium can't be absorbed without calcitriol).

Other factors regulating PTH secretion. Although serum calcium concentration's the most important regulator of PTH secretion, other factors can stimulate or inhibit PTH release. Beta-adrenergic catecholamines, prostaglandins, steroids, and several drug classes help increase PTH. Adenosine 3':5'-cyclic phosphate (cyclic AMP), found throughout the body, works with PTH to permit its action on the target cell. Alpha-adrenergic catecholamines, colchicine, vinblastine, and probenecid inhibit PTH.

Calcitonin activity. Although the thyroid gland's parafollicullar (C) cells produce most body calcitonin, the parathyroid glands contribute a small portion. A polypeptide, calcitonin counterbalances PTH by lowering serum calcium levels. In response to hypercalcemia, the glands increase calcitonin output, which inhibits bone

Continued on page 72

Parathyroid Disorders

Calcium: The key to bone formation and growth

The body's most abundant mineral, calcium plays a key role in many physiologic processes. It ensures neuromuscular integrity by altering cell membrane permeability, thus regulating nerve and cardiac cell threshold potentials. It also aids neurotransmitter release from nerve endings, assists in muscle contraction, promotes hormonal stimulus and secretion, and contributes significantly to blood clotting. By regulating enzyme activity, calcium also affects cellular metabolism.

The bones and teeth contain about 99% of the body's calcium; soft tissues and extracellular fluid contain about 1%.

Calcium regulation. Parathyroid hormone (PTH), vitamin D, and calcitonin regulate the serum calcium level through their effects on target organs (the GI tract, kidneys, and bone).

Serum calcium levels normally range from 8.5 to 10.5 mg/dl (4.5 to 5.2 mEq/liter). Serum contains three calcium forms:
• nondiffusible, protein-bound calcium (about 50% of total serum calcium)
• diffusible, free, physiologically active ionized calcium (about 45% of total serum calcium)
• diffusible, nonionized calcium that's complexed or combined with anions, such as phosphate, sulfate, carbonate, and citrate (about 5% of total serum calcium).

Calcium's distribution among these forms depends on serum protein concentration (with a subnormal serum albumin concentration, the reported total serum calcium may be falsely depressed), serum pH, and serum phosphate levels (as phosphate levels rise, ionized calcium levels fall).

Serum calcium levels also depend on bone activity. Bone tissue continually changes—osteoblasts form new bone, while osteoclasts resorb or demineralize older bone. Young metabolic bone contains only small calcium amounts; older structural bone contains most calcium. The parathyroid glands direct calcium release from older bone. For example, with a low serum calcium level, PTH increases osteo-
Continued

Continued

resorption. When the serum calcium level decreases, so does calcitonin output. Calcitonin reaches its peak action in less than an hour, altering serum calcium levels much more quickly than does PTH. Calcitonin's rapid action significantly reduces acute calcium excess, although it can't sustain this effect in prolonged hypercalcemia.

Hypercalcemia. Defined as a serum calcium level above 10.5 mg/dl, hypercalcemia most commonly stems from hyperparathyroidism. Other possible causes include:
• increased calcium intake, from increased dietary intake or calcium supplementation
• increased GI absorption of calcium, from vitamin D intoxication, sarcoidosis and other granulomatous diseases, or milk-alkali syndrome
• decreased urinary excretion of calcium, from use of drugs such as lithium and thiazide diuretics, milk-alkali syndrome, or conditions producing decreased glomerular filtration
• increased bone resorption from spinal cord injury, immobilization, thyrotoxicosis, vitamin A intoxication, Paget's disease, or cancers with direct skeletal involvement
• Addison's disease
• acromegaly.
(*Note:* Hemoconcentration and an elevated serum albumin level can falsely increase serum calcium levels. Also, signs and symptoms mimicking those of true hypercalcemia can occur from increased ionized calcium levels, without total serum calcium elevation.)

Hypocalcemia. Characterized by a serum calcium level below 8.5 mg/dl, hypocalcemia usually results from hypoparathyroidism and other conditions that disable calcium-regulating mechanisms, such as:
• decreased intestinal absorption, from decreased calcium intake, steroid administration, or chronic diarrhea
• decreased ionized calcium, from hemodilution, alkalosis, or citrated blood administration
• increased calcium loss, from increased urinary loss and body fluid exudate loss
• increased calcitonin levels, from supplemental calcitonin administration, medullary thyroid cancer, or acute pancreatitis
• hyperphosphatemia
• hypomagnesemia
• cardiopulmonary bypass
• use of drugs such as plicamycin and edetate disodium (EDTA).

Assessment
Clues from the patient's history and physical examination may suggest parathyroid dysfunction resulting in a calcium excess or deficit. The patient's chief complaint may vary from muscle weakness and tremors to seizure. Let the patient's responses to your questions guide your history taking. Be sure to investigate his past medical history and his family and social history as well as his present illness.

Parathyroid Disorders

Calcium: The key to bone formation and growth
Continued

clastic activity, stimulating bone breakdown and, thus, calcium release. But phosphate's also released; because of phosphate's reciprocal relationship with calcium, the serum phosphate level must decrease before the serum calcium level can rise. To maintain the serum calcium level, PTH increases renal phosphate excretion. The serum calcium level then rises as the serum phosphate level drops.

Calcitonin release, stimulated by an increased calcium level, inhibits or depresses osteoclastic activity and bone resorption, thus inhibiting calcium release.

Calcium absorption. Ingested in foods such as milk and dairy products, fruits, vegetables, and grain products, calcium must be broken down from the complex to the soluble ionized form for intestinal absorption. Gastric acid increases calcium's solubility and facilitates intestinal absorption. Only about 30% of ingested calcium becomes absorbed—primarily in the duodenum and proximal jejunum, through active and passive mechanisms. Active absorption, requiring a vitamin D metabolite, predominates.

Various factors affect intestinal calcium absorption. Decreased vitamin D, magnesium (which competes with calcium for absorption), small intestine fats, a high-fiber diet, and the aging process decrease absorption. Phosphate deficiency, increased vitamin D and PTH levels, hypocalcemia, pregnancy, and lactation increase absorption.

Both absorbed calcium (secreted via bile into the intestinal lumen) and unabsorbed calcium undergo fecal excretion. Although the kidneys also excrete calcium, about 98% of the filtered calcium becomes reabsorbed. In the proximal tubule, calcium reabsorption accompanies sodium transport. Consequently, extracellular fluid volume, which regulates sodium reabsorption, also regulates calcium reabsorption there.

Selected laboratory tests

Serum parathyroid hormone (PTH)
Helps assess for hyperparathyroidism and hypoparathyroidism

Implications of abnormal results:
Above-normal value suggests hyperparathyroidism; below-normal value suggests hypoparathyroidism.

Nursing considerations:
• Normal values depend on calcium level (some laboratories graph calcium level against PTH level to determine abnormality).
• Test results must be correlated with other findings and with patient's signs and symptoms.

Serum calcium
Assesses for hypercalcemia and hypocalcemia

Implications of abnormal results:
Above-normal value may indicate hypercalcemia; below-normal value may indicate hypocalcemia.

Nursing considerations:
• Serum calcium occurs in both bound and ionized forms. Serum calcium value reflects total of these forms.
• Because nearly half of serum calcium binds to protein, serum albumin level should be measured simultaneously for accurate serum calcium determination. If patient has abnormal albumin value, serum calcium value must be corrected by adding 1 mg/dl calcium for every 1 g/dl albumin decrease below normal.
• Ionized serum calcium level more reliably indicates parathyroid dysfunction than does total serum calcium level. Ratio of ionized to total serum calcium rises above normal with primary hyperparathyroidism.
• Value may decrease with citrated blood administration (citrate binds with calcium).

Serum phosphate
Assesses inorganic serum phosphate level; helps detect hyperparathyroidism and hypoparathyroidism

Implications of abnormal results:
Above-normal value may indicate hypoparathyroidism; below-normal value may indicate hyperparathyroidism.

Nursing considerations:
• Diet can affect test results.
• Values vary throughout the day, peaking at midnight and dropping to lowest level at 8 a.m.
• Have patient fast before sample collection (serum phosphate level falls after meals in response to increased insulin secretion and intracellular phosphate shift).

Sulkowitch's test (urine calcium)
Qualitatively measures urine calcium level; assesses for hyperparathyroidism and hypoparathyroidism

Implications of abnormal results:
Above-normal level suggests hyperparathyroidism. Below-normal level suggests hypoparathyroidism.

Nursing considerations:
• Test may be performed as single random urine specimen or as 24-hour urine collection.
• The doctor may order a low-calcium diet 1 to 3 days before specimen collection to avoid false elevation resulting from high dietary calcium intake. However, some doctors don't advise dietary changes because they believe that a patient with hyperparathyroidism may have a normal urine calcium level on a low-calcium diet but an above-normal level on his standard diet.

Tubular reabsorption of phosphate (TRP)
Helps diagnose primary hyperparathyroidism

Implications of abnormal results:
A reabsorption level below 77% suggests primary hyperparathyroidism.

Nursing considerations:
• Test requires simultaneous blood sample and urine specimen collection.
• Values vary with age, diet, and hormone function.
• Patient must fast before test.
• Tell patient to discard the first morning urine and collect the second.
• Spot urine test requires only about 30 ml.

Urinary cyclic AMP
Assesses for PTH dysfunction

Implications of abnormal results:
Above-normal value suggests hyperparathyroidism; below-normal value suggests hypoparathyroidism.

Nursing considerations:
• Test involves 24-hour urine collection.
• Serum sample may be drawn simultaneously for calcium measurement.
• Test proves unreliable in patients with compromised renal function or with hypercalcemia from an ectopic tumor that produces PTH-like substance.

Because the parathyroid glands can't be palpated, percussed, or auscultated, your physical examination will involve only inspection.

For specific information on evaluating a patient for parathyroid dysfunction, see pages 75 through 79 and pages 84 through 86.

Continued on page 74

Parathyroid Disorders

How vitamin D promotes bone growth

Vitamin D and its metabolites, vitamin D_2 (ergocalciferol) and D_3 (cholecalciferol) have been identified as sterol hormones, with metabolism and mechanisms of action similar to other steroid hormones'.

Vitamin D_2, used to fortify dairy products, derives from ultraviolet radiation of the plant sterol ergosterol. Vitamin D_3 derives mainly from the skin via ultraviolet radiation of 7-dehydrocholesterol.

Vitamin D maintains conditions favoring bone mineralization, increasing serum calcium and phosphate levels by facilitating GI absorption of these minerals. The vitamin D form that promotes intestinal absorption undergoes complex synthesis (see flowchart), beginning with a precursor form in the skin and ending with renal production of 1,25-dihydroxycholecalciferol (1,25[OH]$_2$D$_3$; calcitriol).

Dietary vitamin D_2, used in margarine and cereals, can also be synthesized to produce calcitriol. A potent vitamin D form, calcitriol works in the small intestine to stimulate calcium transport across the mucosal wall into the capillaries.

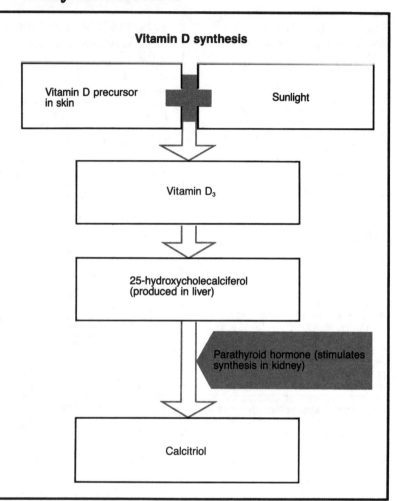

Vitamin D synthesis

Vitamin D precursor in skin + Sunlight → Vitamin D_3 → 25-hydroxycholecalciferol (produced in liver) ← Parathyroid hormone (stimulates synthesis in kidney) → Calcitriol

Continued

Diagnostic studies. Differential diagnosis will help confirm or rule out a parathyroid disorder or determine its underlying cause. See *Selected laboratory tests,* page 73, to review tests typically ordered to evaluate parathyroid function. Other laboratory studies that may be performed include the following:

• *Ellsworth-Howard excretion test (PTH infusion test).* After I.V. administration of PTH extract, hourly urine specimens are collected for phosphorus measurement. This test aids diagnosis of hypoparathyroidism, especially psuedohypoparathyroidism.

• *Calcitonin stimulation test.* The doctor may order this test, which uses pentagastrin and calcium gluconate, if he suspects medullary thyroid cancer (a disease affecting parathyroid function).

Other studies that help assess parathyroid function include computed tomography (CT), ultrasonography, esophagography, parathyroid thermography, thyroid scan, or thyroid angiography (which may include selective venous catheterization).

Hyperparathyroidism

Although the cause of spontaneous parathyroid hyperfunction remains unknown, the disorder can be classified as primary, secondary, or tertiary hyperparathyroidism.

Parathyroid Disorders

Primary hyperparathyroidism involves faulty PTH regulation by one or more parathyroid glands—the normal serum calcium feedback mechanism malfunctions, permitting autonomous PTH production and release. Studies suggest primary hyperparathyroidism can stem from any of the following:

• benign adenoma of one parathyroid gland (approximately 80% of cases)
• genetic factors
• cancer
• neck radiation
• parathyroid hyperplasia
• multiple endocrine neoplasia (MEN), Type I or II (for more information on MEN, see Chapter 6).

Primary hyperparathyroidism occurs much more commonly in women (especially postmenopausal women) than in men, with onset typically between ages 35 and 65.

Secondary hyperparathyroidism reflects compensatory PTH hypersecretion in response to defective calcium homeostasis, such as in chronic renal disease, rickets, osteomalacia, and intestinal malabsorption syndromes.

Tertiary hyperparathyroidism describes the evolution of secondary hyperparathyroidism into primary hyperparathyroidism. This can occur from prolonged compensatory stimulation to an enlarged gland, which then develops autonomous function.

All three hyperparathyroidism types lead to hypercalcemia and hypophosphatemia. Hypercalcemia fails to inhibit parathyroid activity, and the continuing hypercalcemia (not the excess PTH) results in functional and/or structural target organ changes. Signs and symptoms reflect these changes. For example, as urine calcium and phosphorus levels increase, the kidneys fail to concentrate urine, polyuria develops, and renal calculi form, possibly leading to urinary obstruction and/or infection. Bone resorption causes calcium loss, triggering bone demineralization that results in bone pain from pathologic fractures or cystic bone disease (osteitis fibrosa cystica).

Hyperparathyroidism can be acute and severe (when serum calcium levels exceed 15 mg/dl) or chronic and moderate (when serum calcium levels range from 12 to 15 mg/dl).

Assessment

When taking the history of a patient with suspected hyperparathyroidism (hypercalcemia), be sure to ask about thiazide drug use and vitamin D and calcium intake, all of which can produce hypercalcemia. (Extremely high vitamin D doses can lead to severe hypercalcemia, as can excessive calcium intake.) A history of renal calculi suggests hypercalcemia.

Also take a thorough family history—primary hyperparathyroidism occurs in conjunction with several familial MEN syndromes. Ask if the patient has any blood relatives who've had metabolic bone disease, intractable peptic ulcer disease, neck surgery, endocrine tumors, hypercalcemia, or renal calculi. Suspect primary hyper-

Continued on page 76

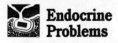
Parathyroid Disorders

Hyperparathyroidism—*continued*

parathyroidism in any mother of an infant with severe neonatal tetany.

Key signs and symptoms. Depending on whether the disorder's acute or chronic, the patient with hyperparathyroidism may lack symptoms or have obvious systemic problems, such as weakness, weight loss, fatigue, headache, and depression. With an asymptomatic patient, the disorder may be discovered only during a routine serum calcium analysis. With gradual symptom onset over several years, the patient may complain of renal colic pain. Some patients have a rapid symptom onset, with marked hypercalcemia, bone pain, pathologic fracture, and weight loss. (To review hypercalcemia signs and symptoms, see *Assessing hyperparathyroidism.*)

Besides the history, general inspection will provide the most valuable clues to hyperparathyroidism. Palpation, percussion, and auscultation usually reveal little, depending on the patient and the disease stage. Use the following common findings, classified by body system, as an assessment guide:

Renal system. Excessive PTH production causes increased serum and renal tubular calcium reabsorption. At the same time, PTH blocks proximal tubular phosphate reabsorption, resulting in hypophosphatemia. Renal response to PTH also includes decreased acid excretion and increased potassium, bicarbonate, and phosphate excretion, leading to urinary alkalosis, metabolic acidosis, and hypokalemia.

Calcium accumulation can result in renal calculi or parenchymal calcification; either condition may lead to extensive renal damage and failure. Signs and symptoms include renal colic, back pain, hematuria, and renal calculi passage.

Skeletal system. Normally, bone surface osteoblastic activity exceeds osteoclastic activity. With hyperparathyroidism, however, osteoblastic activity diminishes gradually as PTH action increases bone resorption, leading to calcium release into the blood. This decalcification may cause bone pain, bone cysts, pathologic fracture, localized jawbone swelling, brown tumors (large cystic lesions, also called osteoclastomas), or generalized osteoporosis. The jaw, hands, spine, and skull most readily reveal these structural changes, with demineralized areas appearing on X-ray in advanced disease stages.

GI system. PTH stimulates renal synthesis of calcitriol. This, in turn, triggers dietary calcium absorption in the duodenum and upper jejunum. The resulting hypercalcemia may cause anorexia, nausea, vomiting, and constipation. Hypercalcemia increases serum gastrin, which stimulates increased gastric hydrochloric acid secretion, possibly causing peptic ulcer. Cholelithiasis may result from increased biliary calcium concentration, promoting formation of calcium bilirubinate stones. Pancreatitis may also occur, although its mechanism remains unclear.

Cardiovascular system. Hypercalcemia slows cardiac function by increasing myocardial contractility and decreasing automaticity. An EKG will reveal a shortened QT interval, a slightly prolonged PR

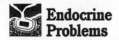
Parathyroid Disorders

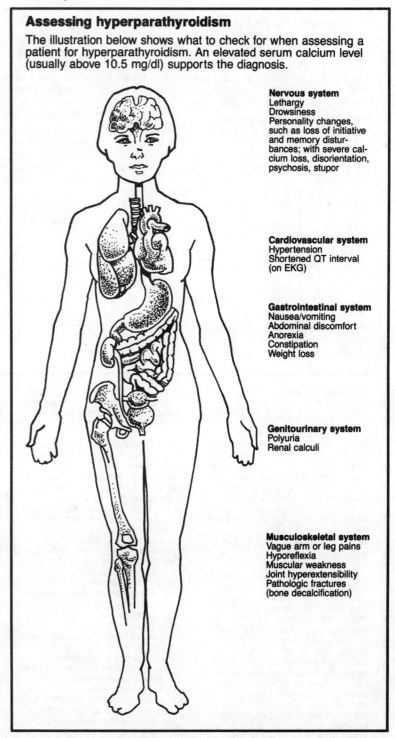

Assessing hyperparathyroidism

The illustration below shows what to check for when assessing a patient for hyperparathyroidism. An elevated serum calcium level (usually above 10.5 mg/dl) supports the diagnosis.

Nervous system
Lethargy
Drowsiness
Personality changes, such as loss of initiative and memory disturbances; with severe calcium loss, disorientation, psychosis, stupor

Cardiovascular system
Hypertension
Shortened QT interval (on EKG)

Gastrointestinal system
Nausea/vomiting
Abdominal discomfort
Anorexia
Constipation
Weight loss

Genitourinary system
Polyuria
Renal calculi

Musculoskeletal system
Vague arm or leg pains
Hyporeflexia
Muscular weakness
Joint hyperextensibility
Pathologic fractures
(bone decalcification)

interval and QRS complex, absent ST segment, and a widening T wave. Myocardial sensitivity to digitalis increases with hypercalcemia, potentiating the drug's effects. Heart failure associated with vascular damage and kidney disease may occur. Most patients with hyperparathyroidism also have hypertension, possibly from elevated plasma renin.

Neuromuscular system. As the calcium level increases above normal (to at least 12 mg/dl), neuromuscular depression sets in. First,

Continued on page 79

Parathyroid Disorders

Phosphate and phosphatic disorders

Phosphate, an important bone component, promotes production of the vitamin D metabolite calcitriol, which facilitates intestinal absorption of phosphate and calcium. Depressed serum phosphate increases calcitriol production; elevated serum phosphate inhibits production.

Phosphate also serves these other key functions:
• aids cellular metabolism (particularly in red blood cells) by
combining with lipids to form phospholipids—substances that make up the cell membrane
• combines with nucleic acids, forming phosphoproteins—essential to the mitochondrial electron transport system
• assists in the intermediary metabolism of carbohydrates, fats, and proteins
• helps produce 2,3-diphosphoglycerate (2,3-DPG), which promotes hemoglobin's oxygen-carrying capacity
• forms high-energy phosphate bonds in adenosine triphosphate (ATP); these bonds power virtually all physiologic activity.

The skeleton, where phosphate deposition and release take place, stores about 85% of the body's phosphate; soft tissues and cells contain the rest.

The serum phosphate level normally ranges from 2.5 to 4.5 mg/dl, fluctuating with pH changes, glucose metabolism, and certain hormonal influences, and varying inversely with serum calcium changes. (*Note:* Serum phosphorus may be measured instead of serum phosphate to determine the total concentration of inorganic phosphates.)

Found in most foods, phosphate's especially abundant in red meats, fish, poultry, milk and milk products, eggs, nuts, and legumes. The body absorbs about 80% of ingested phosphate, excreting unabsorbed phosphate in the feces.

The kidneys primarily regulate total body phosphate by filtering it at the glomerulus and reabsorbing it in the proximal convoluted tubule, loop of Henle, and the nephron's distal portion.

Parathyroid hormone (PTH) promotes bone resorption and draws phosphate from bone. At the same time, it increases renal phosphate excretion, allowing ionized serum calcium levels to increase. Vitamin D helps PTH to draw phosphate from bone and increases intestinal phosphate absorption.

Hyperphosphatemia. This occurs when serum phosphate levels exceed 4.5 mg/dl. It typically occurs with acute or chronic renal insufficiency or hypoparathyroidism. As renal function fails, glomerular filtration suffers, leading to diminished phosphate excretion. Serum phosphate levels then rise. Hypomagnesemia and hypoparathyroidism decrease renal phosphate excretion. Hyperphosphatemia can also arise from overcorrected hypophosphatemia.

Hyperphosphatemia's physiologic effects stem from the reciprocal relationship between calcium and phosphate. As the serum phosphate level increases, phosphate combines with free calcium, causing a decreased ionized serum calcium level. This accelerates PTH production, resulting in secondary hyperparathyroidism and an elevated serum calcium level. Serum phosphate and calcium levels then rise, which causes the combination product—calcium phosphate—to increase until calcium phosphate crystals form. These crystals, insoluble in plasma, precipitate, producing metastatic calcifications in the brain, eyes, gums, skin, joints, lungs, myocardium, blood vessels, and heart valves. Bone demineralization and dissolution occur as parathyroid stimulation continues, resulting in osteomalacia, osteitis fibrosa, and osteosclerosis.

Intervention. Phosphate-binding preparations, particularly aluminum hydroxide gels, help correct hyperphosphatemia. Calcium and vitamin D supplements also help reduce the serum phosphate level. Advise the patient to avoid phosphate-rich foods, including whole grain cereals, cream, hard cheeses, nuts, dried fruits and vegetables, and specialty meats (such as kidney, brain, and liver).

Hypophosphatemia. This disorder occurs when the serum phosphate level drops below 2.5 mg/dl. However, total body phosphate depletion may not take place until the level drops below 1.0 mg/dl, indicating severe hypophosphatemia. Causes of hypophosphatemia include:
• chronic alcoholism
• diabetic ketoacidosis
• decreased phosphate intake and absorption, such as from starvation, vomiting or diarrhea, phosphate-poor I.V. hyperalimentation, malabsorption syndrome, small-bowel or pancreatic disease, gastrectomy, and ingestion of aluminum or magnesium hydroxide antacids
• increased renal phosphate losses, such as from Fanconi's syndrome, Wilson's disease, nephrotic syndrome, hypokalemia, hypomagnesemia, hyperparathyroidism, or thiazide diuretic use
• transcellular shifts, as with I.V. glucose or insulin administration, I.V. hyperalimentation, and respiratory alkalosis.

Signs and symptoms appear when the serum phosphate level falls below 2.0 mg/dl. These changes result from decreased ATP production and/or decreased 2,3-DPG, which lead to altered cellular function and reduced cellular oxygenation.

The patient may have any of the following signs and symptoms:
• anemia
• decreased white blood cell bactericidal activity
• thrombocytopenia and hemorrhage, from platelet dysfunction and destruction
• generalized muscle weakness, lassitude, malaise, tremors, paresthesias, ataxia, and waddling gait
• reddish-brown urine, from urinary myoglobin excretion
• increased creatine phosphokinase levels
• memory loss, reduced attention span, confusion, disorientation, and convulsions
• absent or decreased reflexes, impaired sensory function, and ascending paralysis, from spinal cord dysfunction
• unequal pupil size, ptosis, vertigo, nystagmus, nasal speech, and dysarthria, from cranial nerve palsy
• metabolic acidosis, from renal changes
• osteomalacia, bone pain, and pathologic and pseudofractures, from bone calcium loss
• anorexia, nausea, vomiting, and other nonspecific GI complaints
• reduced cardiac output, from ATP reduction
• dysrhythmias, from ischemia
• rapid, shallow respirations, from decreasing tidal volume and vital capacity
• hepatic encephalopathy and portal hypertension, from impaired hepatic function.

Intervention. Mild hypophosphatemia usually responds to increased dietary phosphate intake, such as from dairy products. Moderate hypophosphatemia usually improves with oral phosphate supplements. A patient with severe hypophosphatemia may require I.V. phosphate therapy.

To prevent hypophosphatemia, the doctor may advise your patient to take aluminum phosphate antacids (such as Phosphojel) or cimetidine (Tagamet) instead of phosphate-binding antacids.

Parathyroid Disorders

Hyperparathyroidism—*continued*

lethargy and weakness develop, followed by depressed reflexes, muscle hypotonicity, confusion, and coma as calcium levels rise progressively higher.

Central nervous system. Hyperparathyroidism may produce apathy; personality changes; depression; irritability; mood swings; or unusual, unexplainable emotions.

Diagnostic studies. An above-normal serum calcium level (usually defined as higher than 10.5 mg/dl) serves as the key finding in hyperparathyroidism (normal serum calcium levels range from 8.5 to 10.5 mg/dl [4.5 to 5.2 mEq/liter]). The doctor usually diagnoses the disorder from elevated serum calcium levels (preferably confirmed by at least three measurements) and from the patient's signs and symptoms.

Other diagnostic findings suggesting hyperparathyroidism include:
• above-normal urinary cyclic AMP level (in patients with normal renal function)
• above-normal serum PTH level, as measured by radioimmunoassay (inconclusive by itself, this finding must be evaluated in conjunction with serum calcium concentration and the patient's clinical condition).

Tests that help determine or localize the cause of hyperparathyroidism include esophagography, thyroid scans, parathyroid thermography, ultrasonography, CT scan, and thyroid angiography (which may include selective venous catheterization). X-rays help assess bone or renal calcification.

Planning
Before determining your nursing care plan, develop the nursing diagnosis by identifying your patient's problem or potential problem, then relating it to its cause. Possible nursing diagnoses for a patient with hyperparathyroidism include:
• fluid volume, alteration in (deficit); related to hypercalcemia
• anxiety; related to possible surgery
• cardiac output, alteration in (decreased); related to hypercalcemia
• comfort, alteration in (renal colic); related to renal calculi development
• activity intolerance; related to weakness and fatigue
• knowledge deficit; related to newly diagnosed disease
• memory deficit; related to hypercalcemia
• thought processes, alteration in; related to hypercalcemia.

The sample care plan on page 80 shows expected outcomes, nursing interventions, and discharge planning for one nursing diagnosis listed above. However, you'll want to tailor each care plan to your patient's needs.

Intervention
Treatment of hyperparathyroidism may include surgery and/or medical measures.

Surgery. Candidates for parathyroidectomy include those with primary hyperparathyroidism affecting the kidneys or extensive bone

Continued on page 80

Parathyroid Disorders

Sample nursing care plan: Hyperparathyroidism

Nursing diagnosis	Expected outcomes
Fluid volume, alteration in (deficit); related to hypercalcemia	The patient will: • maintain adequate urine output. • lack signs and symptoms of renal calculi.
Nursing interventions • Discuss disorder and treatment plan with patient and family. • Encourage patient to drink at least 3,000 ml of fluids/day (unless contraindicated)—especially fluids that promote acidic urine, such as cranberry and prune juice. • Encourage ambulation or other activity to prevent urinary stasis. • If indicated, strain urine for calculi. • Monitor fluid intake and output. • Assess for signs and symptoms of dehydration, such as dry mucosa, decreased skin turgor, excessive thirst, and decreased urine output.	**Discharge planning** • Reinforce with patient and family what doctor has told them about patient's disease and care plan. • Advise patient when to seek medical care. • Arrange for follow-up care, if indicated.

Hyperparathyroidism—*continued*

areas or causing peptic ulcer or pancreatitis. Surgical removal of three parathyroid glands with subtotal resection of the fourth may be performed for primary hyperplasia of all four glands or for one or more parathyroid adenomas (one intact parathyroid gland provides sufficient function to prevent hypoparathyroidism).

In the most common parathyroidectomy procedure, the doctor first identifies all four glands (using biopsy, if necessary), removes diseased tissue, then marks the remaining glands or tissue remnants with nonabsorbable sutures to aid identification should recurrent hyperparathyroidism necessitate further surgery. If the doctor can't identify abnormal parathyroid tissue, he'll probably perform hemithyroidectomy for a potential intrathyroid lesion.

For a patient with parathyroid glands located mediastinally (usually in the superior chest cavity, attached to the thymus or mediastinal fat pad), surgical treatment may include a mediastinotomy.

If your patient's had surgery for hyperparathyroidism, watch for these potential complications:
• hemorrhage (because of the highly vascular area surrounding the parathyroid glands)
• infection
• laryngeal paralysis or voice loss or change (from damage to the nearby recurrent laryngeal nerve)
• respiratory distress secondary to tracheal edema or compression by an overly constrictive occlusive dressing
• difficulty in swallowing, secondary to edema or pressure on the esophagus
• transient hypoparathyroidism. This occurs in most postparathyroidectomy patients (acute hypocalcemia or tetany may arise 1 to 4 days after surgery). Signs and symptoms of postoperative hypoparathyroidism, which stem from neuromuscular irritability, may include:
—nervousness and irritability

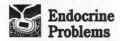
Parathyroid Disorders

Parathyroidectomy

Parathyroidectomy serves as the only curative treatment for primary hyperparathyroidism. After making a transverse cervical incision, the surgeon explores the exposed area to identify the parathyroid gland (or glands). The superior glands prove easier to locate than the inferior glands. (The illustration below shows the surgeon locating the left inferior parathyroid gland.) Before removing the gland, he'll take a tissue sample for biopsy to ensure correct gland identification.

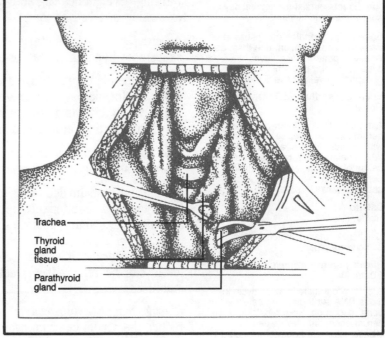

Trachea

Thyroid gland tissue

Parathyroid gland

—tetany (as indicated by circumoral and carpopedal spasm and numbness)
—muscle cramps (prolonged and painful, as in a charley horse)
—dysphagia
—hyperactive tendon reflexes
—tonic and clonic convulsions
—laryngeal stridor
—prolonged QT interval on EKG
—positive Chvostek's and Trousseau's signs.

Medical intervention. The doctor will order medical therapy for a patient too ill to risk surgery or for one with nonresectable cancer. Medical measures aim to reduce serum calcium to a safe (although not necessarily normal) level. Specific measures will depend on the patient's serum calcium level and on whether the condition's acute and severe or chronic and moderate.

Acute, severe hypercalcemia—a life-threatening condition—requires early detection and prompt treatment focusing on rehydration, mobilization, and drug or dietary calcium restrictions.

To reverse dehydration—which results from impaired renal concentrating ability, nausea, and vomiting—the doctor may order I.V. saline solution or isotonic sodium sulfate as well as diuresis (with furosemide or ethacrynic acid). These measures help increase urinary calcium excretion, thus decreasing the exchangeable calcium pool and reducing serum calcium concentration. Saline solution promotes calcium excretion because calcium clearance accompanies

Parathyroid autotransplantation

For some patients with hyperparathyroidism from enlarged parathyroid glands, the doctor may recommend parathyroid autotransplantation—gland removal and partial replacement in another body region. Besides reducing parathyroid mass, autotransplantation permits normal calcium homeostasis.

The procedure involves two stages. First, the doctor performs a total parathyroidectomy, preserving parathyroid tissue by freezing. Later, if necessary, he autografts parathyroid tissue to the patient's forearm muscles or another site. This allows easy removal of some pieces using local anesthesia should hyperparathyroidism recur.

A normal serum calcium level (revealing normal parathyroid function) and high serum parathyroid hormone levels in the antecubital vein draining the graft bed indicate successful autotransplantation.

Continued on page 82

Parathyroid Disorders

Drugs that decrease serum calcium levels

Phosphates
Route: I.V., oral (as with Phospho-Soda or Neutra-Phos), rectal (as with a Fleet enema)

Phosphates reduce serum calcium levels by inhibiting bone resorption and promoting bone mineral accretion. Effects persist for several days after the last administration.

Because phosphates can cause extraskeletal calcification, use them cautiously in patients with severe hypercalcemia, azotemia, or serum phosphate levels above 3 mg/dl.

Edetate disodium (EDTA)
Route: I.V.

Although EDTA helps reduce the serum calcium level by combining with calcium to form a stable excretable chelate, it's rarely used now because of its transient effects and nephrotoxicity and because it may cause severe I.V. pain.

Calcitonin
Route: I.V., I.M.

Calcitonin potently inhibits osteoclastic bone resorption.

Plicamycin (mithramycin)
Route: I.V.

A cytotoxic antibiotic, plicamycin inhibits RNA synthesis and osteoclastic bone resorption. Serum calcium and serum phosphate levels usually decrease within 24 hours of a single I.V. dose, with effects persisting for about 1 week. Plicamycin also helps manage long-term severe hypercalcemia.

Because plicamycin can cause marked thrombocytopenia, use it cautiously in patients with compromised hematologic status or primary hyperparathyroidism (because of the potential need for surgery). Monitor for early signs of liver, kidney, or bone marrow toxicity.

Steroids
Route: Parenteral or oral

Steroids such as hydrocortisone reduce the serum calcium level by inhibiting vitamin D- and vitamin A-induced bone resorption and reducing vitamin D's effect on intestinal calcium absorption.

Indomethacin
Route: Oral

With hypocalcemia caused by cancer, indomethacin helps inhibit increased bone resorption (resulting from cancer-induced prostaglandin excess).

Hyperparathyroidism—*continued*

sodium clearance; furosemide inhibits tubular reabsorption of calcium and helps maintain diuresis.

Mobilization helps reverse the effects of immobility, including an increased bone resorption rate (particularly in a patient with a preexisting high resorption rate). Encourage standing or assisted walking—weight-bearing activities that prove more beneficial than exercising in a bed or chair.

As ordered, restrict dietary calcium and all drugs that cause or exacerbate hypercalcemia; for example, thiazides and vitamin D.

Hypercalcemia may increase a patient's sensitivity to digitalis. For a hypercalcemic patient receiving digitalis, the doctor may reduce the digitalis dose as a precaution. Monitor the patient's EKG while instituting antihypercalcemic measures.

Additional measures to reduce the serum calcium level include drug therapy (see *Drugs that decrease serum calcium levels*).

Once serum calcium decreases to a reasonably safe level, the patient may require a maintenance regimen including furosemide or ethacrynic acid, sodium chloride tablets, at least 3,000 ml of fluids a day, and, if necessary, magnesium and potassium supplements. Daily monitoring of serum calcium, magnesium, and potassium levels can be replaced by weekly checks once the calcium level stabilizes.

Chronic, moderate hypercalcemia necessitates drug therapy to help reduce the serum calcium level and correct hypercalcemia's cause. Besides the drugs listed at left, therapy may include estrogen, which decreases bone resorption as well as the serum calcium level. Unless the patient has a family history of uterine or breast cancer, expect the doctor to order maintenance doses of unconjugated estrogen. Alpha- and beta-adrenergic blockers and cimetidine may also help treat chronic, moderate hypercalcemia.

Evaluation

Base your evaluation on the expected outcomes listed on the nursing care plan. To determine if the patient's improved, ask yourself the following questions:
• Can the patient maintain an adequate fluid intake and volume?
• Does he have signs and symptoms of dehydration?
• Does he have signs and symptoms of renal calculi?
• Does he know which fluids to drink to help keep his urine acidic?

The answers to these questions will help you evaluate your patient's status and the effectiveness of his care. Keep in mind that these questions stem from the sample nursing care plan on page 80. Your questions may differ.

Hypoparathyroidism

In this disorder, PTH secretion or peripheral PTH action decreases. The patient has a subnormal serum calcium level and an above-normal serum phosphate level, along with signs and symptoms of neuromuscular hyperactivity (such as tetany). Hypoparathyroidism can be iatrogenic, idiopathic, or functional.

Continued on page 84

Parathyroid Disorders

Magnesium and magnesium disorders

Magnesium, an abundant cation, potently affects cellular metabolism and other body functions. Its intracellular effects:
• aid phosphate transfer reactions that break down adenosine triphosphate (ATP) to release energy and adenosine diphosphate (ADP)
• regulate the sodium/potassium pump to control intracellular potassium concentration
• aid binding of messenger RNA to ribosomes during protein synthesis
• take part in glucose metabolism.

Magnesium also helps regulate serum calcium concentration via its effects on parathyroid hormone (PTH) secretion; acts as a neuromuscular sedative by blocking or decreasing acetylcholine release at nerve endings; and aids in growth, wound healing, temperature regulation, myocardial activity, and immunocompetence.

Bone contains about half the body's magnesium. Other intracellular structures contain about 49%; extracellular fluid contains about 1%.

Serum magnesium levels, which normally range from 1.8 to 3.0 mg/dl (1.5 to 2.5 mEq/liter), don't necessarily reflect total body magnesium. Below-normal serum albumin hemodilution can falsely reduce serum magnesium concentration.

Magnesium's supplied by many foods, particularly leafy green vegetables, whole grains, nuts, meats, fish, peanut butter, milk, tea, eggs, cheese, beans, and bananas. Daily magnesium intake averages 20 to 40 mEq. Of this amount, the body absorbs about 30%, primarily through the proximal small intestine.

Intestinal magnesium absorption takes place by two routes—one that competes with calcium for absorption and another that's independent of calcium absorption. Magnesium homeostasis depends mainly on the kidneys, which filter about 70% to 80% at the glomerulus and reabsorb about 20% to 30% in the proximal convoluted tubule.

PTH and hypomagnesemia can increase proximal tubular magnesium reabsorption. The following factors can decrease absorption, promoting magnesium loss:
• use of drugs, such as gentamicin, tobramycin, and carbenicillin
• hormone therapy, such as with thyroxine, calcitonin, growth hormone, or aldosterone
• physiologic processes, such as renal vasodilation and hypercalcemia
• increased sodium intake.

Hypermagnesemia. This condition, marked by serum magnesium levels above 2.5 mEq/liter, can arise from reduced magnesium excretion (most commonly from severe renal failure) or increased magnesium intake (usually from frequent use of magnesium-containing antacids or laxatives). Increased intake also occurs through prolonged, excessive magnesium supplementation, frequent magnesium sulfate enemas, and excessive magnesium in I.V. hyperalimentation fluids. Addison's disease (adrenocortical insufficiency), lithium administration, and myxedema have also been linked with hypermagnesemia.

Signs and symptoms usually don't appear until the serum magnesium level rises above 4 mEq/liter. Findings may include the following:
• weak to absent deep-tendon reflexes
• muscle paralysis
• hypotension, flushing, sweating, heat sensation, bradycardia, heart block, cardiac arrest
• drowsiness, lethargy
• respiratory muscle paralysis and apnea
• excessive thirst, nausea and vomiting
• reduced PTH secretion.

Intervention. Treatment aims to eliminate the cause as well as relieve signs and symptoms. Anticholinesterase drugs help reverse neuromuscular depression. Withholding magnesium supplements and administering fluid and calcium salts help correct the underlying cause. A

patient with renal failure may need dialysis.

Hypomagnesemia. Defined as a serum magnesium concentration below 1.5 mEq/liter, hypomagnesemia occurs much more commonly than hypermagnesemia. The disorder can result from:
• reduced magnesium intake, such as from protein-calorie malnutrition, starvation, and prolonged I.V. therapy without magnesium supplementation
• decreased intestinal absorption, as from malabsorption syndromes, bowel resection, or intestinal disorders
• increased urinary excretion, as from diuresis, renal disorders, hyperaldosteronism, hyperthyroidism, and hypocalcemia
• excessive body fluid loss, as from chronic diarrhea, draining fistulas, prolonged nasogastric suctioning, prolonged lactation, and burns.

Other causes include multiple transfusions with citrated blood, cardiopulmonary bypass pump use, and acute pancreatitis.

Signs and symptoms, which typically appear only when the serum magnesium level falls below 1 mEq/liter, mainly involve the central nervous system, neuromuscular system, GI tract, and cardiovascular system. Hyperirritability may lead to mental status changes, insomnia, auditory and visual hallucinations, confusion, agitation, nervousness, personality changes, delirium, depression, and psychosis.

Neuromuscular excitability may cause muscle twitching, grimaces, paresthesias, tremors, leg cramps, hyperactive reflexes, positive Babinski's reflex, alternating muscle relaxation and contraction, muscle clonus, choreiform movements (involuntary jerky, irregular movements of the face, trunk, arms, and legs), athetoid movements (similar to choreiform movements but slower, with more twisting and writhing), respiratory stridor, dysphagia, nystagmus, papilledema, positive Chvostek's sign, seizures, overt tetany, and generalized spasticity.

GI problems, usually resulting from concomitant hypokalemia, may include nausea, vomiting, anorexia, diarrhea, and abdominal distention. Hypokalemia and/or hypocalcemia may cause such cardiovascular changes as dysrhythmias (for example, supraventricular and ventricular tachycardias or premature atrial and ventricular beats).

Intervention. Treatment depends on the disorder's severity and the patient's clinical condition. An asymptomatic patient usually responds to increased dietary magnesium intake, through such foods as nuts, cereals, refined sugars, seafood, meats, legumes, and vegetables. Magnesium-containing antacids or oral magnesium supplements also help increase magnesium levels. In acute hypomagnesemia requiring emergency treatment, expect the doctor to order parenteral or I.V. magnesium sulfate.

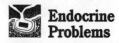
Parathyroid Disorders

Pseudohypoparathyroidism

A rare hereditary disorder, pseudohypoparathyroidism causes hypocalcemia, hyperphosphatemia, and a diminished target organ response to parathyroid hormone (PTH). The patient may have an above-normal serum PTH level.

Signs and symptoms, which typically appear at about age 8, include a round face; short stature; a short, thick neck; obesity; decreased intelligence; and subcutaneous calcification. Bony anomalies also occur, including shortened metacarpals, metatarsals, and phalanges (most commonly of the ring finger).

Pseudohypoparathyroidism requires the same treatment as hypoparathyroidism—lifelong vitamin D and calcium supplements. Long-term nursing goals focus on educating the patient about his drug and dietary regimens and providing emotional support.

Hypoparathyroidism—*continued*

Iatrogenic hypoparathyroidism. The most common type, this may result from any surgical procedure involving the anterior neck, such as thyroidectomy or neck irradiation. Parathyroid tissue removal or damage can also result in hypoparathyroidism, as can interrupted parathyroid blood supply.

Parathyroid gland removal leads to:
• decreased bone resorption
• decreased renal phosphate excretion with an increased serum phosphate level, decreased calcitriol, and decreased intestinal calcium absorption
• increased renal calcium excretion relative to the serum calcium concentration.

Idiopathic hypoparathyroidism. This broad category includes early-onset and late-onset hypofunction. Genetic causes and congenital parathyroid gland absence (as in DiGeorge's syndrome) cause early-onset disorders. Researchers have identified organ-specific antibodies circulating to parathyroid and adrenal tissue in patients with genetic early-onset disorders. Pernicious anemia, ovarian failure, and autoimmune thyroiditis also take place in some early-onset patients.

(*Note:* Early-onset idiopathic hypoparathyroidism also goes by the terms multiple endocrine deficiency, autoimmune, candidiasis [MEDAC] syndrome; and juvenile familial endocrinopathy, also known as hypoparathyroidism, Addison's disease, and mucocutaneous candidiasis [HAM] syndrome).

Late-onset disorders tend to occur sporadically and don't involve circulating glandular antibodies. The cause of parathyroid gland destruction hasn't been identified.

Functional hypoparathyroidism. Patients who have had long-term hypomagnesemia (including those with GI malabsorption disorders or alcoholism) may experience this hypoparathyroidism form. PTH release (and probably peripheral PTH action) depend on magnesium. Therefore, low magnesium levels may partly account for absent PTH action on the normal target tissues and subsequent hypocalcemia.

Assessment

Signs and symptoms of hypoparathyroidism result from hypocalcemia. Neuromuscular problems are the most important findings. By increasing neuromuscular excitability, hypocalcemia causes problems, such as tetany. Early symptoms include muscle cramps and tingling and numbness around the mouth and on the tips of fingers and toes. (Cramps resulting from reduced calcium typically last several minutes, with residual muscle soreness after cramping.) Hyperreflexia may also occur.

In later disease stages, the patient may experience tetany. Prodromal paresthesia and facial, arm, and leg muscle spasms typically precede a tetany attack. The hands, forearms, and, less commonly, the feet may contort in a characteristic pattern, with thumb ad-

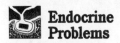

Parathyroid Disorders

Eliciting hypocalcemia signs

Chvostek's sign. To elicit this sign, tap the patient's facial nerve just in front of the earlobe and below the zygomatic arch; or alternatively, between the zygomatic arch and the corner of the mouth. A positive response (indicating latent tetany) ranges from simple mouth-corner twitching to twitching of all facial muscles on the side tested. Simple twitching may be normal in some patients. However, a more pronounced response usually indicates a positive Chvostek's sign.

Trousseau's sign. Test for this sign by inflating a blood pressure cuff to a level above systolic pressure. Maintain this pressure for at least 2 minutes while observing the patient's hand for a carpal spasm. Then deflate the cuff. A spasm lasting 5 to 10 seconds after cuff deflation means a positive response. (An instantly disappearing spasm may be normal.)

The most reliable sign of latent tetany, Trousseau's sign should be tested serially.

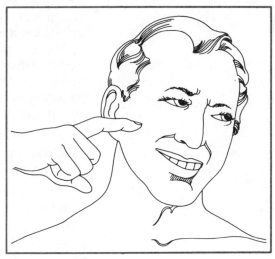

Chvostek's sign

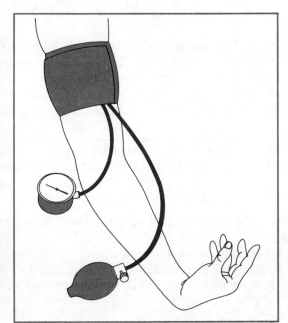

Trousseau's sign

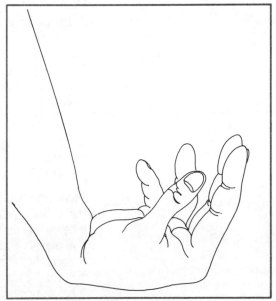

Carpal spasm in Trousseau's sign

duction followed by metacarpophalangeal joint flexion, interphalangeal joint extension, and wrist and elbow joint flexion (see *Eliciting hypocalcemia signs*).

Tetany may trigger a cyclic reaction: Anxiety resulting from the tetany attack leads to hyperventilation, which, in turn, causes hypocapnia and alkalosis. This worsens the hypocalcemia that triggered the tetany. The patient may also have seizures and laryngeal spasms, so be sure to assess for and maintain a patent airway.

Other signs and symptoms of hypoparathyroidism, classified by body system, include the following:

Continued on page 86

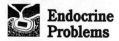
Parathyroid Disorders

Hypoparathyroidism—*continued*

Central nervous system. Expect personality changes ranging from irritability, agitation, and anxiety to depression, delirium, frank psychosis, and, in some cases, intellectual impairment. Papilledema, elevated cerebrospinal fluid pressure, and neurologic signs mimicking cerebral tumor may occur. A patient with chronic hypoparathyroidism may undergo intracranial calcification, particularly in the basal ganglia, leading to parkinsonian-like symptoms.

GI system. Hypocalcemia can cause nausea, vomiting, abdominal pain, and constipation or diarrhea. Such symptoms may mimic an acute abdominal disorder.

Cardiovascular system. Decreased calcium levels can cause cardiac dysrhythmias, decreased contractility, and reduced cardiac output. (*Note:* Suspect hypocalcemia in a patient who complains of pain when you take his blood pressure.)

Visual system. Lens calcification leads to cataract formation that persists despite hypocalcemia correction.

Integumentary system. Skin changes most commonly occur with idiopathic or chronic hypoparathyroidism. The skin becomes dry, scaly, coarse, pigmented, and infection-prone. Patchy alopecia and loss of eyebrow, eyelash, axillary, and pubic hair may occur. Fingernails and toenails become brittle and deformed, developing horizontal ridges.

You may elicit signs of latent tetany—Chvostek's and Trousseau's signs—on physical examination. Keep in mind that although some individuals normally have a positive Chvostek's sign, only a hypocalcemic patient has a positive Trousseau's sign.

Diagnostic studies. Laboratory findings associated with hypoparathyroidism include:
• below-normal serum calcium level
• above-normal serum phosphate or serum phosphorus level
• normal or slightly above-normal serum alkaline phosphatase level
• normal serum magnesium level
• below-normal serum PTH level
• below-normal or absent Sulkowitch's test value for urinary calcium excretion
• below-normal urinary creatinine level.

You may also detect a prolonged QT interval on EKG.

Depending on the suspected cause of hypoparathyroidism, the doctor may order other studies, such as X-rays, CT scans, and ultrasound.

Planning
Before determining your nursing care plan, develop the nursing diagnosis by identifying your patient's problem or potential problem, then relating it to its cause. Possible nursing diagnoses for a patient with hypoparathyroidism include:
• knowledge deficit; related to calcium and vitamin D supplement therapy

Parathyroid Disorders

- gas exchange, impaired; related to laryngeal spasms (a result of tetany)
- injury, potential for (tetany); related to hypocalcemia
- anxiety; related to tetany
- injury, potential for; related to I.V. calcium administration
- noncompliance; related to long-term calcium and vitamin D supplement therapy.

The sample care plan below shows expected outcomes, nursing interventions, and discharge planning for one nursing diagnosis listed above. However, you'll want to tailor each care plan to your patient's needs.

Intervention

Treatment goals for the patient with hypoparathyroidism focus on preventing tetany and correcting hypocalcemia. Acute hypocalcemia calls for I.V. calcium gluconate or calcium chloride administration. Long-term management involves vitamin D and oral calcium therapy.

Continued on page 88

Sample nursing care plan: Hypoparathyroidism

Nursing diagnosis	Expected outcomes
Knowledge deficit; related to calcium and vitamin D supplement therapy	The patient will: • show that he understands the rationale for calcium and vitamin D supplement therapy. • plan a diet high in calcium and vitamin D and low in phosphate. • show that he understands the route, dose, schedule, and potential adverse effects of his supplemental medications.
Nursing interventions • Discuss disorder, treatment, and care plan with patient and family. • Discuss the importance of long-term management and follow-up care (especially periodic serum calcium testing). • Instruct patient about foods high in calcium and vitamin D, such as dairy products, green leafy vegetables, salmon, egg yolks, and shrimp. Advise him to avoid high-phosphate foods, such as spinach, rhubarb, and asparagus. • Discuss medication supplements, including their purpose, doses, administration routes, and adverse effects. • Advise patient to take calcium supplements with or after meals, and, if possible, to chew tablets to a fine powder rather than swallowing them whole. If indicated, suggest that he take oral calcium with orange juice to enhance calcium absorption. • Discuss the use of phosphate binders, such as Amphojel, before meals to help reduce phosphate absorption and raise serum calcium levels. • Discuss the importance of taking vitamin D to ensure calcium absorption and mobilization from bone and to promote phosphate excretion.	**Discharge planning** • Reinforce patient instructions. • Arrange for a dietitian to discuss dietary planning with patient and family. • Make sure patient and family can recognize tetany signs and symptoms. • Advise patient when to seek medical care. • Arrange for follow-up care, if indicated.

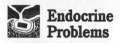
Parathyroid Disorders

Parenteral calcium supplements

Calcium gluconate (10%)
(93 mg calcium; 4.6 mEq)
Route and dose
I.V.: 20 to 30 ml in 100 ml dextrose 5% in water over 10 to 15 minutes, or as ordered
I.M.: As ordered
Nursing considerations
• Supplement may cause hypotension.
• Avoid I.M. route in infants because of possible abscess formation.

Calcium gluceptate (1.1 g/5 ml)
(90 mg calcium; 4.5 mEq)
Route and dose
I.V.: 10 to 15 ml in 100 ml dextrose 5% in water over 10 to 15 minutes, or as ordered
I.M: As ordered
Nursing considerations
• Supplement may cause hypotension, metallic taste, or transient arm and leg tingling.
• Check for local irritation at injection site.

Calcium chloride (10%)
(272 mg calcium; 13.6 mEq)
Route and dose
I.V.: 5 to 10 ml in 100 ml dextrose 5% in water over 10 to 15 minutes, or as ordered
I.M.: Not used
Nursing considerations
• Supplement may cause hypotension and local and GI irritation.
• Don't administer with sodium bicarbonate—a precipitate may form.
• Check for tissue sloughing from I.V. infiltration.

Hypoparathyroidism—*continued*

To help prevent or manage tetany, the doctor will focus interventions on:
• providing an emergency airway if laryngeal spasms occur
• administering I.V. calcium to elevate the serum calcium level. (*Note:* When administering I.V. calcium, don't use saline solution, which promotes calcium and sodium excretion, thus worsening hypocalcemia. Also avoid bicarbonate solutions, which cause precipitation.)

Definitive therapy requires vitamin D administration, which should begin as soon as possible. Vitamin D preparations include ergocalciferol (vitamin D_2), dihydrotachysterol (Hytakerol), calcifediol (Calderol), and calcitriol (Rocaltrol). Before vitamin D therapy takes effect, the doctor may want to maintain serum calcium for several days at levels sufficient to prevent tetany. Combined oral and intermittent I.V. calcium administration help accomplish this goal.

Treatment goals for chronic hypoparathyroidism include alleviating signs and symptoms and avoiding vitamin D intoxification.

Because vitamin D promotes intestinal calcium absorption, make sure the patient has a total (dietary and supplemental) intake of at least 1 g of calcium daily. Oral calcium preparations include calcium gluconate tablets, calcium glubionate (Neo-Calglucon), calcium lactate, and calcium carbonate (Titralac, Os-Cal).

When administering oral calcium supplements, watch for signs of adverse effects, such as acid-base imbalance. Instruct the patient to chew the calcium tablet into fine particles rather than swallowing it whole. A high milk or milk-product intake can serve as a supplement to or substitute for oral calcium.

The patient receiving calcium and vitamin D supplement therapy should have his serum calcium and serum phosphorus (or phosphate) levels checked frequently to monitor for hypercalcemia. If your patient must continue such therapy after discharge, warn him that he risks irreversible renal impairment if he fails to comply with the monitoring schedule.

Evaluation
Base your evaluation on the expected outcomes listed on the sample nursing care plan. To determine if the patient's improved, ask yourself the following questions:
• Does the patient understand the rationale for calcium and vitamin D supplement therapy?
• Can he plan a nutritionally sound diet that's high in calcium and vitamin D but low in phosphate?
• Does he know how to take his supplemental medications and how to identify their adverse effects?
• Does he know the signs and symptoms of tetany and when to seek medical care?

The answers to these questions will help you evaluate your patient's status and the effectiveness of his care. Remember that these questions stem from the sample nursing care plan on page 87. Your questions may differ.

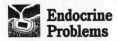
Parathyroid Disorders

Self-Test

1. Bone resorption refers to:
a. bone formation through mineral deposition b. bone formation through osteoblastic activity c. mineral migration from bone into blood d. mineral migration from blood into bone

2. All of the following regulate serum calcium levels except:
a. serum protein concentration b. calcitonin c. vitamin D d. parathyroid hormone (PTH)

3. A reduced serum calcium level leads to:
a. a PTH increase, causing bone demineralization b. a PTH decrease, causing bone demineralization c. a PTH increase, causing bone formation d. a PTH decrease, causing bone formation

4. Hypophosphatemia signs and symptoms may include all of the following except:
a. thrombocytopenia b. muscle weakness c. increased cardiac output d. rapid, shallow respirations

5. Magnesium plays an important role in calcium metabolism by modifying:
a. PTH secretion b. calcitonin secretion c. vitamin D metabolism d. glucose metabolism

6. Bone demineralization accompanying hyperparathyroidism results from:
a. bone resorption b. bone mineralization c. decreased osteoclastic activity d. increased osteoblastic activity

7. Treatment of the patient with acute, severe hypercalcemia (resulting from hyperparathyroidism) includes all of the following except:
a. mobilization by encouraging weight-bearing activity
b. rehydration by administering I.V. dextrose solutions c. dietary calcium restriction d. diuresis by administering furosemide or ethacrynic acid

8. If your patient's recovering from a parathyroidectomy, assess him for all of the following except:
a. hypocalcemia (tetany) b. voice loss or change c. tracheal edema d. renal calculi

9. A hypoparathyroid patient may have all of the following signs and symptoms except:
a. a positive Trousseau's sign b. nausea and vomiting c. a shortened QT interval on EKG d. tetany

10. Which of the following measures *won't* the doctor order for a hypoparathyroid patient?
a. phosphate supplementation b. I.V. calcium supplementation c. oral calcium supplementation d. vitamin D supplementation

Answers (page number shows where answer appears in text)
1. **c** (page 70) 2. **a** (page 70) 3. **a** (pages 72-73) 4. **c** (page 78) 5. **a** (page 83) 6. **a** (page 75) 7. **b** (pages 81-82) 8. **d** (page 80) 9. **c** (page 86) 10. **a** (page 87)

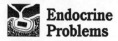

Pancreatic Disorders: Diabetes Mellitus and Hypoglycemia

Marlene M. Ciranowicz, who wrote this chapter, is an independent nursing consultant. She received her BSN from Gwynedd Mercy College, Gwynedd Valley, Pa., and her MSN from the University of Pennsylvania, Philadelphia.

In this chapter, we'll focus on the most prevalent disorders resulting from pancreatic endocrine dysfunction—hyperglycemia (diabetes mellitus) and hypoglycemia. These disorders, which involve cell clusters called the islets of Langerhans, rank as the most common cause of endocrine dysfunction. (For information on pancreatic *exocrine* dysfunction, see the NURSEREVIEW section on "Gastrointestinal Problems.") Before reviewing these disorders in depth, read this brief summary of pancreatic endocrine function (see also *Reviewing pancreatic structure and function*).

Reviewing pancreatic structure and function

The pancreas, a fish-shaped gland measuring 3″ to 4″ (7.6 to 10.2 cm), lies behind the stomach. It performs both endocrine and exocrine functions.

Endocrine function results from the *islets of Langerhans,* scattered groups of specialized alpha, beta, and delta cells. Alpha cells secrete glucagon; beta cells secrete insulin; delta cells secrete somatostatin. (Also secreted by the hypothalamus and the GI tract, somatostatin may inhibit insulin and glucagon secretion.) The ductless islets release these hormones interstitially for eventual absorption into the bloodstream, where they modify blood glucose regulation.

Exocrine function results from the activity of enzyme-producing cells (*acini*) distributed throughout the pancreas. These cells secrete digestive enzymes, releasing them through pancreatic ducts into the gastrointestinal tract, where they aid digestion. (See the NURSEREVIEW section on "Gastrointestinal Problems" for more information on these enzymes.)

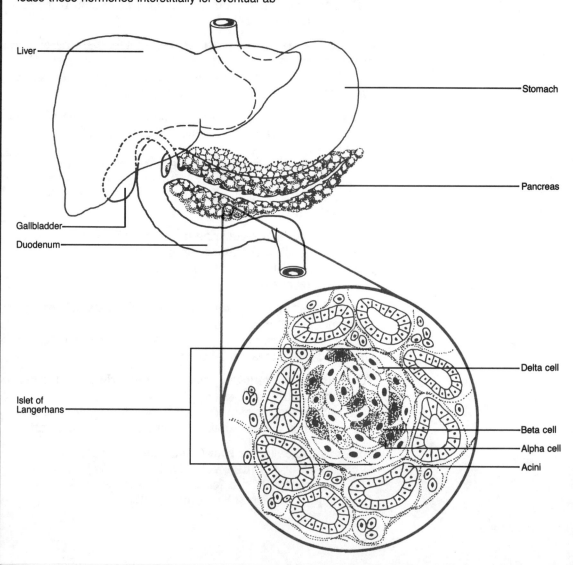

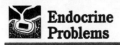
Pancreatic Disorders

Continued on page 92

Blood glucose regulation

Insulin, glucagon, epinephrine, glucocorticoids (cortisol), and growth hormone all help regulate blood glucose levels. Increased blood glucose levels stimulate secretion of insulin, the main regulatory hormone. Besides reducing blood glucose levels, insulin increases glucose uptake and glycogen synthesis and inhibits glycogenolysis and gluconeogenesis.

Decreased blood glucose levels (as with hypoglycemia, exercise, and high protein intake) stimulate secretion of:
• glucagon, which increases glycogenolysis and gluconeogenesis
• epinephrine, which increases glycogenolysis and reduces peripheral glucose uptake
• glucocorticoids, which increase gluconeogenesis and decrease peripheral glucose uptake
• growth hormone, which reduces peripheral glucose uptake.

Reviewing common terms

Glycogenesis: Glycogen formation from carbohydrates

Glycogenolysis: Glycogen conversion into glucose 6-phosphate, and free glucose liberation in liver

Glycolysis: Glucose breakdown into pyruvic or lactic acid

Gluconeogenesis: Glucose formation from noncarbohydrates

Lipogenesis: Conversion of fatty acids and glycerol, or excess carbohydrates and protein, into fat (usually for adipose tissue storage)

Lipolysis: Triglyceride hydrolysis into fatty acids and glycerol

Pancreatic hormone production. The pancreas produces two major hormones, insulin and glucagon. *Insulin,* a protein produced in the islets' beta cells, has two release patterns. The pancreas releases a small amount (measured as the basal rate) continuously and a larger amount (measured as the bolus rate) in response to a stimulus, such as an increased glucose level. Once released, insulin speeds glucose transport from the bloodstream through cell membranes, thus increasing the glucose available to cells and decreasing the circulating glucose (see *Blood glucose regulation*). The islets produce about 50 units of insulin daily; usually, the pancreas stores about 200 units.

A few cells (such as red blood cells and brain and renal tubule cells) don't need insulin to transport glucose. However, for most cells (and for overall body metabolism), insulin plays a critical role, increasing tissue glycogen storage, enhancing glucose metabolism, and decreasing blood glucose concentration (if necessary, the body can convert stored glycogen to glucose).

Insulin deficiency (as in diabetes mellitus) causes profoundly abnormal carbohydrate, lipid, and protein metabolism. Because the body can't use carbohydrates efficiently without adequate insulin, it begins to metabolize fat. Ketone bodies—intermediate fat metabolism products—accumulate in the blood. Ultimately, abnormal carbohydrate, lipid, and protein metabolism result in pronounced hyperglycemia, osmotic diuresis, severe dehydration, electrolyte imbalance, metabolic acidosis, and severe weight loss.

Insulin excess (as from insulinoma [islet beta cell tumor]) also causes disruptive metabolic effects, particularly hypoglycemia.

The islets' alpha cells produce *glucagon* in response to low blood glucose levels. Glucagon stimulates liver gluconeogenesis and glycogenolysis and thus increases the blood glucose level (see *Reviewing common terms*).

Glucagon and insulin secretion depend on blood glucose levels. Increased blood glucose levels trigger insulin secretion and suppress glucagon secretion. Decreased blood glucose levels trigger glucagon release and suppress insulin secretion.

Primary glucagon imbalance occurs rarely, from such disorders as familial hyperglucagonemia and glucagonoma (islet alpha cell tumor). Most commonly, elevated glucagon levels appear with diabetes mellitus. Because insulin inhibits glucagon secretion, its absence or deficiency allows continued glucagon secretion even with hyperglycemia.

Carbohydrate metabolism. Glucose, a 6-carbon monosaccharide, serves as the body's main energy source. Blood glucose derives from:
• conversion of ingested carbohydrates by digestive tract enzyme activity
• metabolic conversion of noncarbohydrate liver and kidney sources
• breakdown of hepatic and peripheral glycogen (major glucose storage forms).

Insulin and glucagon, as discussed above, chiefly regulate glucose levels. However, several other hormones also affect glucose levels

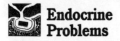
Pancreatic Disorders

Pancreatic hormones

Hormone	Releasing/inhibiting stimulus	Primary target site	Primary effects
Insulin (from beta cells)	High blood glucose concentration, nutritional need, food ingestion, neural impulses (such as from stress), somatostatin, and other factors	Most body tissues	• Increases lipogenesis (promotes fat storage) • Increases glycogen synthesis • Stimulates protein synthesis (promotes tissue building) • Decreases blood glucose level • Decreases glycogenolysis • Decreases gluconeogenesis
Glucagon (from alpha cells)	Low blood glucose concentration, nutritional need, food ingestion, neural impulses (such as from stress), somatostatin, and other factors	Liver, adipose tissue	• Increases blood glucose level • Increases gluconeogenesis • Increases glycogenolysis • Increases lipogenesis
Somatostatin (from delta cells)	Food ingestion, neural impulses (such as from stress)	Pancreatic alpha and beta cells, pituitary gland	• Reduces insulin and/or glucagon secretion • Impedes growth hormone release

Continued

and contribute to normal carbohydrate metabolism. For example, growth hormone, secreted by the anterior pituitary lobe, raises glucose levels by promoting glucose formation from fat and protein. Cortisol and similar 11-oxysteroids, secreted by the adrenal cortex, have the same effect. Epinephrine and thyroxine increase blood glucose levels by stimulating glycogen's conversion to glucose.

Here's how carbohydrate metabolism works: Food ingestion causes a modest blood glucose rise, triggering pancreatic insulin secretion and release. Insulin stimulates cellular glucose absorption and promotes glucose conversion to storage forms. In the liver, insulin increases glucose conversion to glycogen (glycogenesis) and thus inhibits hepatic glycogen breakdown to glucose. The liver and peripheral tissues normally store ingested glucose as glycogen. In the muscles, insulin enhances protein synthesis and amino acid storage and promotes glucose conversion to glycogen or fat. In adipose tissue, insulin helps synthesize triglyceride, inhibiting its breakdown to free fatty acids and glycerol. Hepatic and peripheral glucose uptake depend on prompt insulin secretion and on normal tissue responsiveness to insulin.

In the fasting state, the body derives energy from the stored sources discussed above. As blood glucose levels fall, insulin secretion diminishes and glucagon concentration rises. Without dietary carbohydrates (the body's preferred energy source), glucagon stimulates glucose formation from protein catabolized in the liver and kidneys (gluconeogenesis) and from hepatic glycogen breakdown (glycogenolysis). In adipose tissue, glucagon stimulates triglyceride breakdown to free fatty acids and glycerol (lipolysis). In the muscles, glucagon breaks down protein into amino acids (proteolysis).

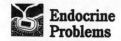
Pancreatic Disorders

Assessment

The history and physical examination of a patient with pancreatic endocrine dysfunction focus on evaluating for signs and symptoms of glucose excess or deficit. Check for classic diabetes mellitus signs and symptoms, including:

• polyuria
• polydipsia
• polyphagia
• weight loss
• fatigue.

In some cases, the patient may have signs and symptoms of hypoglycemia, including:
• adrenergic signs and symptoms (nervousness, hunger, and diaphoresis)
• neuroglycopenic (neurologically induced) signs and symptoms (altered level of consciousness, headache, and blurred vision).

In a few patients, premature myocardial infarction or peripheral vascular disease provides the first clue to diabetes mellitus.

As always, investigate the patient's chief complaint, present illness, past medical history, family history, and social history. Use your patient's chief complaint and his signs and symptoms to guide your assessment; but remember that these may be vague, suggesting various disorders. Make sure you take a detailed health history, which may give clues to your patient's disorder. The health history may be the *only* clue to a blood glucose alteration in a patient without suggestive physical findings. The history also plays an important role in identifying the hypoglycemia or hyperglycemia type.

Because you can't palpate, percuss, or auscultate the pancreas, you'll rely on *inspection* for physical evidence of glucose excess or deficit. Your findings will depend on the severity of the patient's blood glucose alteration at the examination time. Keep in mind, however, that physical examination proves important even when the patient has no acute signs of hypoglycemia or hyperglycemia— your findings may reveal evidence of associated complications.

Diagnostic studies. A simple blood glucose analysis can confirm an altered blood glucose level. The doctor may order a blood glucose analysis with the patient in a fed or fasting state. If this test proves inconclusive, he may order glucose tolerance testing. If he identifies or suspects *hypoglycemia,* he may order serum insulin and C-peptide tests to help identify the hypoglycemia type. If he identifies *hyperglycemia* (usually a chronic dysfunction), he may order further tests to monitor blood glucose levels. These tests include urine glucose and acetone tests, hemoglobin A_{1c} (glycohemoglobin) tests, and blood glucose self-monitoring. (See *Selected laboratory tests,* pages 94 and 95, and the information under "Diabetes mellitus" for details on these tests.)

If your patient's receiving insulin to treat diabetes mellitus, the doctor may order an insulin antibody test, a radioimmunoassay technique that detects antibodies to injected insulin. Most insulin

Continued on page 95

Pancreatic Disorders

Selected laboratory tests

Fasting blood glucose

Measures blood glucose level after 12- to 14-hour fast; diagnoses diabetes mellitus and helps assess hypoglycemia and monitor diabetes mellitus control

Implications of abnormal results:
Above-normal level on more than two occasions confirms diabetes mellitus; deviations also occur with such disorders as acute pancreatitis, myocardial infarction, chronic liver disease, and gastrectomy. Below-normal level usually indicates hypoglycemia, possibly stemming from such disorders as hyperinsulinism, insulinoma, adrenal insufficiency, and hypopituitarism.

Nursing considerations:
• Fasting reduces blood glucose levels, stimulating glucagon release. Glucagon increases blood glucose levels by accelerating glycogenolysis, stimulating gluconeogenesis, and inhibiting glycogen synthesis. Normally, insulin secretion inhibits this glucose increase. In a diabetic patient, absent or deficient insulin causes persistently high glucose levels.
• Make sure patient has fasted before drawing blood (he can resume eating after test).
• Observe patient for signs and symptoms of glucose alteration.
• Ensure proper sample timing.
• Modify diabetes therapy according to appropriate guidelines.

Two-hour postprandial blood glucose

Helps screen for diabetes mellitus in patient with suggestive signs and symptoms or when results of fasting blood glucose test suggest diabetes; helps monitor diabetes drug or diet therapy

Implications of abnormal results:
Above-normal level suggests diabetes mellitus but may also occur with pancreatitis, Cushing's syndrome, pheochromocytoma, hyperlipoproteinemia, sepsis, gastrectomy with dumping syndrome, and other disorders. Below-normal level suggests hypoglycemia, possibly stemming from such disorders as hyperinsulinism, insulinoma, adrenal insufficiency, and hypopituitarism.

Nursing considerations:
• Advise patient to eat balanced diet or one containing 100 g carbohydrate before test, then to fast for 2 hours. Test usually takes place 2 hours after meal or glucose load administration.
• Instruct patient to avoid smoking and strenuous exercise after pretest meal.

Oral glucose tolerance test (OGTT)

Measures insulin response to glucose challenge; helps diagnose diabetes mellitus (especially in borderline cases) and hypoglycemia (also helps identify hypoglycemia type)

Implications of abnormal results:
• Above-normal value in 2-hour sample and another sample taken up to 2 hours later suggests diabetes mellitus. Below-normal value indicates reactive hypoglycemia.

Nursing considerations:
• Test measures carbohydrate metabolism after ingestion of challenge glucose dose. The body absorbs this dose rapidly, causing blood glucose levels to rise and peak in 30 to 60 minutes. The pancreas responds by secreting more insulin, causing glucose levels to return to normal after 2 to 3 hours. Test monitors blood and urine glucose levels during this period to assess insulin secretion and the body's ability to metabolize glucose. To aid diagnosis of hypoglycemia and malabsorption syndrome, levels may be monitored for an additional 2 to 3 hours.
• If indicated, instruct patient to maintain high-carbohydrate diet for 3 days and then to fast for 10 to 16 hours before test.
• Advise patient not to smoke, drink coffee or alcohol, or exercise strenuously for 8 hours before or during test.
• Make sure patient recognizes hypoglycemia symptoms—weakness, restlessness, nervousness, hunger, and sweating—and tell him to report such symptoms immediately.
• After drawing fasting blood glucose sample and collecting urine specimen (if ordered), administer oral glucose test load and record ingestion time. Encourage patient to drink entire glucose solution within 5 minutes.
• Draw blood sample 30 minutes, 1 hour, 2 hours, and 3 hours after giving loading dose. Collect urine specimens at the same intervals (if ordered).

I.V. glucose tolerance test

Measures insulin response to glucose challenge; helps diagnose diabetes mellitus and hypoglycemia

Implications of abnormal results:
Failure to achieve fasting glucose levels within 2 to 3 hours suggests diabetes mellitus, although this response may also result from fever, stress, old age, inactivity, carbohydrate deprivation, neoplasm, cirrhosis, or a steroid-producing endocrine disease. Below-normal value indicates fasting hypoglycemia.

Nursing considerations:
• Test measures blood glucose after patient receives I.V. infusion of glucose 50% solution over 3 or 4 minutes. Draw blood samples 30 minutes, 1 hour, 2 hours, and 3 hours after infusion. After an immediate glucose peak of 300 to 400 mg/dl (accompanied by glycosuria), the normal glucose curve falls steadily, reaching fasting levels within 1 to 1¼ hours.
• Test provides alternative to flat OGTT curves resulting from hypopituitarism, hypoparathyroidism, or Addison's disease.
• Test has the following disadvantages:
—provides less reliable results than OGTT
—doesn't consistently diagnose mild diabetes.

Cortisone glucose tolerance

Measures insulin response to corticosteroids; helps diagnose diabetes mellitus

Implications of abnormal results:
Value that rises approximately 20 mg/dl above that of standard OGTT after 2 hours indicates probable diabetes mellitus in some persons with only minimally decreased carbohydrate intolerance.

Nursing considerations:
• Test can be used to assess patients with borderline carbohydrate-tolerance deficiencies and those with strong familial predisposition to diabetes who present a normal OGTT curve.
• Patient must eat high-carbohydrate diet for 3 days before test.
• Patient receives oral cortisone acetate or prednisone 8½ and 2 hours before standard OGTT. (Cortisone promotes glyconeogenesis and may accentuate carbohydrate intolerance in latent or mild diabetes).

Tolbutamide tolerance

Measures insulin secretion from pancreatic beta cells and certain tumors after I.V. tolbutamide infusion; helps diagnose insulinoma, rule out functional hyperinsulinism, and detect mild diabetes mellitus

Implications of abnormal results:
Because blood glucose levels normally decrease rapidly after tolbutamide infusion and return to pre-test levels in 1½ to 3 hours, abnormal insulin secretion can be detected indirectly by monitoring blood glucose levels. In hyperinsulinism, blood glucose levels mirror those found in normal persons. In insulinoma, glucose levels drop sharply and may take up to 3 hours to return to pre-test levels. In diabetes mellitus, initial blood glucose drop occurs more slowly, with prolonged return to pre-test levels.

Nursing considerations:
• Although this test can help determine the cause of severe hypoglycemia shown by fasting blood glucose test or 2-hour postprandial glucose test, it's contraindicated in patients with fasting blood glucose levels that fall below 50 mg/dl. Be-

Continued

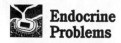
Pancreatic Disorders

Tolbutamide tolerance

continued

cause tolbutamide depresses blood glucose to about half the fasting level, it can cause such patients to develop severe hypoglycemia, leading to seizures and coma.
• Test should not be performed in patients with hypersensitivity to tolbutamide or other sulfonylureas and should be used cautiously in patients with known hypersensitivity to sulfonamides.
• Instruct patient to eat high-carbohydrate diet (150 to 300 g/day) for 3 days before test and then to fast overnight. Also instruct him to avoid smoking during fast and test.
• Alert patient to hypoglycemia symptoms—weakness, restlessness, nervousness, hunger, and sweating—and tell him to report such symptoms immediately.
• After collecting fasting blood glucose sample, administer mixture of 1 g tolbutamide and 20 ml sterile water, as ordered (shake solution to dissolve any crystals). Infuse solution I.V. over 2 or 3 minutes. After infusion, if patient has suspected insulinoma or hyperinsulinism, draw blood samples at 15, 30, 45, 60, 90, 120, 150, and 180 minutes after in-

fusion. If patient has suspected diabetes mellitus, draw blood samples 20 and 30 minutes after infusion.

Serum insulin
Measures serum insulin level; helps determine hypoglycemia cause (such as insulinoma or islet cell hyperplasia) and detects insulin resistance

Implications of abnormal results:
Above-normal level may indicate insulinoma. Above-normal *or* below-normal level may signify diabetes mellitus (level depends on diabetes' cause). *Note:* Results must be correlated with blood glucose measurement.

Nursing considerations:
• Make sure patient has fasted for 10 to 15 hours before test.
• Draw blood glucose sample concomitantly with serum insulin sample.

Serum glucagon
Evaluates patients with suspected glucagonoma (alpha cell tumor) or hypoglycemia from idiopathic glucagon deficiency or pancreatic dysfunction. Test usually takes place concomitantly with serum glucose

and insulin measurements because glucose and insulin levels affect glucagon secretion

Implications of abnormal results:
Markedly above-normal fasting glucagon level suggests glucagonoma. Above-normal level also occurs in diabetes mellitus, acute pancreatitis, and pheochromocytoma. Below-normal level suggests idiopathic glucagon deficiency or hypoglycemia from chronic pancreatitis.

Nursing considerations:
• Instruct patient to fast for 10 to 12 hours before test.
• Make sure patient's relaxed and recumbent for 30 minutes before test.

Plasma C-peptide
Measures blood's C-peptide level; helps differentiate between fasting and pharmacologic hypoglycemia

Implications of abnormal results:
• Above-normal level indicates fasting hypoglycemia; normal level suggests pharmacologic hypoglycemia.

Nursing considerations:
• C-peptide levels correlate strongly with insulin levels.

Continued

preparations (derived from beef or pork pancreases) contain insulin-related peptides as impurities. IgG antibodies form in response to these peptides and complex with subsequent insulin injections, neutralizing insulin's effect. Antibody detection confirms this process as the cause of insulin resistance and suggests the need for a different insulin type.

Other tests that help determine the cause of pancreatic dysfunction include ultrasonography and computed tomography. For information on tests used to monitor blood glucose levels in a patient with confirmed diabetes mellitus (such as hemoglobin A_{1c} testing, urine testing, and blood glucose self-monitoring), see pages 111 to 113.

Diabetes mellitus

Diabetes mellitus represents several chronic, heterogeneous disorders characterized by hyperglycemia and, usually, urinary glucose excretion. Insulin absence or deficiency or inefficient peripheral cell insulin use impairs the body's carbohydrate metabolism. In 1979, the National Diabetes Data Group (through the National Institutes of Health) reclassified diabetes mellitus into the following groups to provide uniform identification criteria (see also *Classifying glucose-intolerance disorders*, page 96):
• Type I: insulin-dependent diabetes mellitus (IDDM); previously called juvenile diabetes
• Type II: non-insulin-dependent diabetes mellitus (NIDDM); previously called adult-onset or maturity-onset diabetes
• Other diabetes mellitus types; previously called secondary diabetes.

Continued on page 96

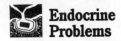
Pancreatic Disorders

Classifying glucose-intolerance disorders

In 1979, the National Diabetes Data Group (NDDG) of the National Institutes of Health proposed new categories of diabetes mellitus and other glucose intolerance–related conditions.

NDDG class	Former terms
DIABETES MELLITUS	
Type I. Insulin-dependent diabetes mellitus (IDDM)	• Juvenile diabetes, juvenile-onset diabetes, ketosis-prone diabetes, unstable or brittle diabetes
Type II. Non-insulin-dependent diabetes mellitus (NIDDM) • Nonobese NIDDM • Obese NIDDM (includes families with autosomal dominant inheritance)	• Adult-onset diabetes, maturity-onset diabetes, ketosis-resistant diabetes, stable diabetes
Other types, including diabetes mellitus associated with certain conditions and syndromes: pancreatic disease; hormonal, drug- or chemical-induced disorders; certain genetic syndromes; insulin receptor abnormalities	• Secondary diabetes
IMPAIRED GLUCOSE TOLERANCE (IGT)	
Nonobese IGT Obese IGT IGT associated with certain conditions and syndromes: pancreatic disease; hormonal, drug- or chemical-induced disorders; insulin receptor abnormalities; certain genetic syndromes	• Asymptomatic diabetes, chemical diabetes, latent diabetes, borderline diabetes, subclinical diabetes
GESTATIONAL DIABETES	
Occurs only during pregnancy	• Gestational diabetes
STATISTICAL RISK CLASSES	
Previous abnormality of glucose tolerance: patients now have normal glucose tolerance but previously had diabetic hyperglycemia or IGT, either spontaneously or in response to a known stimulus; includes former gestational and obese diabetics and others who have had transient hyperglycemia	• Subclinical diabetes, prediabetes, latent diabetes
Potential abnormality of glucose tolerance; includes persons who have never had abnormal glucose tolerance but who are at increased statistical risk for diabetes because of age, weight, race, or family history	• Prediabetes, potential diabetes

Diabetes mellitus—*continued*

Type I diabetes mellitus. Insulin-dependent diabetes mellitus accounts for about 10% of diabetes mellitus cases. It primarily affects young people, although it can arise at any age. This form has an abrupt onset. With rapid beta cell destruction, the patient develops absolute insulin deficiency requiring daily insulin replacement therapy.

The etiology underlying Type I diabetes mellitus remains unknown. Possible factors, all under current investigation, include genetics, viruses, and autoimmunity.

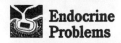

Pancreatic Disorders

• *Genetics.* Many patients with Type I diabetes mellitus have a family history of diabetes. They're also more likely to have certain predisposing genetic patterns that help predict diabetes development. Researchers have linked Type I diabetes mellitus to certain genetic markers in the human leukocyte antigen (HLA) system.

• *Viruses.* Because viral infections may affect the pancreas of a person genetically predisposed to diabetes, researchers continue to investigate a possible link between viruses and Type I diabetes. Antibodies produced after viral infection can attack beta cells, leading to diabetes. The Coxsackie B_4 virus, for instance, has been shown to destroy beta cells. Twenty other viruses have also been linked to Type I diabetes.

• *Autoimmunity.* Because some diabetic patients develop antibodies to pancreatic islet cells, researchers believe an abnormal immune response leads the body to identify pancreatic cells as foreign and destroy them. A defective HLA system can have the same effect.

Type II diabetes mellitus. Non-insulin-dependent diabetes mellitus accounts for about 90% of diabetes cases. It occurs primarily in obese individuals over age 40 who have a strong family history of the disease. However, it can also affect nonobese individuals of any age. It typically has a gradual onset, and causes vague signs and symptoms—beta cells produce some insulin, but not enough to meet the body's needs. The patient may have the disease for many years without knowing it; meanwhile, his body undergoes insidious tissue destruction. Diet, exercise, sulfonylurea (oral hypoglycemic) drugs, and insulin can be used in various combinations to control hyperglycemia.

As with Type I diabetes mellitus, Type II diabetes mellitus has an undefined etiology. The factors implicated in Type I diabetes mellitus don't seem to play a role in Type II. Instead, researchers suspect a beta cell defect and/or a peripheral site defect. A beta cell defect alters insulin secretion, modifying insulin's quantity or quality. A peripheral site defect limits insulin's ability to bind to cell walls— a condition known as *insulin resistance.* Because insulin resistance decreases with weight reduction, researchers believe obesity promotes insulin resistance.

Other diabetes mellitus types. Types I and II diabetes arise spontaneously, not in association with another primary disease. However, in a few patients, diabetes results from another condition or treatment, such as pancreatic disease, hormonal or genetic syndromes, or ingestion of certain drugs or chemicals. These other diabetes types disappear once the precipitating cause has been corrected.

Pathophysiology

Diabetes progresses the same way regardless of the cause or type. Insufficient insulin (either from the beta cells' failure to produce the right amount or quality, or from peripheral cell insulin resistance) leads to altered carbohydrate, protein, and fat metabolism.

Glucose (the body's major energy source) enters the bloodstream from digestion of dietary carbohydrates or through gluconeogenesis and glycogenolysis. It's actively transported to cells that need energy. However, cells can't use glucose without insulin, which in-

Continued on page 98

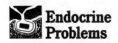
Pancreatic Disorders

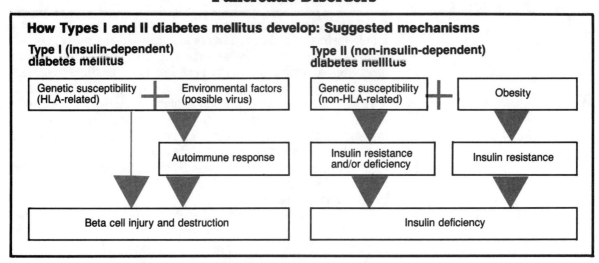

How Types I and II diabetes mellitus develop: Suggested mechanisms

Type I (insulin-dependent) diabetes mellitus

Genetic susceptibility (HLA-related) + Environmental factors (possible virus) → Autoimmune response → Beta cell injury and destruction

Type II (non-insulin-dependent) diabetes mellitus

Genetic susceptibility (non-HLA-related) + Obesity → Insulin resistance and/or deficiency / Insulin resistance → Insulin deficiency

Hyperglycemia: Recognizing classic signs and symptoms

Suspect diabetes mellitus if your patient has the following hyperglycemia signs and symptoms:
• *polyuria* (excessive urination)—from osmotic diuresis caused by excessive blood glucose
• *polydipsia* (excessive thirst)—from polyuria-induced dehydration
• *polyphagia* (excessive hunger)—from increased metabolic needs caused by tissue destruction
• *weight loss and fatigue*—from loss of carbohydrate fuel source and fat and protein depletion to satisfy energy needs.

Diabetes mellitus—*continued*

creases glucose transport through cell membranes. When insulin's unavailable or unusable (as with diabetes mellitus), glucose remains trapped in the blood, with some eventually spilling into the urine. The resulting hyperglycemia causes osmotic diuresis, leading to polyuria, dehydration, and electrolyte imbalances. Pronounced bicarbonate excretion also occurs. With continued osmotic diuresis, cardiac output decreases, followed by hypotension and circulatory collapse.

Meanwhile, glucose-starved cells lack sufficient energy to function. The body attempts to compensate by using protein as an alternate fuel, breaking it down to amino acids from which the liver can form new glucose. Storage glycogen forms begin converting to glucose in an attempt to increase glucose available to cells. (The body can't differentiate between a glucose shortage and an insulin insufficiency.) However, these processes prove ineffective and only worsen hyperglycemia.

The body also uses fat as an alternate fuel source. Unlike protein, fat can be used directly by most cells. However, it's not an efficient cellular fuel and breaks down into two by-products: free fatty acids and glycerol (a glucose substance that exacerbates hyperglycemia). The liver further breaks down free fatty acids into ketone bodies. In Type I diabetes, fat breakdown occurs so quickly that the liver can't handle the excessive ketone bodies. Ketone bodies then spill into the bloodstream, causing ketoacidosis (for further information, see the *Complications* section). In Type II diabetes mellitus, the limited insulin supply allows cells to function, even if only sluggishly. Usually, ketoacidosis doesn't occur.

Assessment

During the history and physical examination, focus on identifying signs and symptoms in these three groups:
• those related directly to elevated blood glucose levels
• those arising from long-term effects of elevated blood glucose levels
• those resulting from disease processes accelerated or exacerbated by diabetes mellitus.

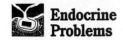
Pancreatic Disorders

Because diabetes mellitus (particularly Type II) may cause no overt signs and symptoms, it may be detected only from a routine examination that reveals hyperglycemia or glycosuria.

History. Begin your assessment by obtaining a thorough history. Typical chief complaints include polyuria, polydipsia, polyphagia, weight loss, and fatigue. Or the patient may complain of weakness, vision changes, frequent skin infections (such as boils, carbuncles, or furuncles), vaginal discomfort or irritation, or dry, itchy skin (see *Hyperglycemia: Recognizing classic signs and symptoms*). Note the severity and duration of the patient's complaints, which may help you identify the diabetes type (Type I diabetes mellitus usually causes pronounced, rapidly developing symptoms; Type II usually leads to vague, long-standing, gradually developing symptoms).

Ask the patient about a past medical history of conditions associated with diabetes mellitus. In particular, note a history of gestational diabetes or the delivery of any baby weighing more than 9 lb (4 kg), recent viral infection, autoimmune dysfunction, other endocrine disorders (particularly thyroid or adrenal disease), and recent stress or trauma. Obtain a thorough drug history because many drugs, such as steroids, can increase blood glucose levels. Note a family history of diabetes mellitus (Type II diabetes mellitus has a strong hereditary component).

When you investigate the patient's social history, assess his nutritional status (particularly his dietary habits) to help evaluate his educational needs as well as his physical condition.

If your patient has previously diagnosed diabetes, determine how well he understands the disease and identify any problems he's encountered. Also find out how successfully he's managed his disease and ask him if he's noticed any symptoms of possible complications.

Physical examination. Perform a thorough physical examination to identify signs of diabetes mellitus and any accompanying complications. If you note signs of acute complications (hypoglycemia, diabetic ketoacidosis, or hyperglycemic hyperosmolar nonketotic coma), notify the doctor immediately and begin interventions as directed (see the *Complications* section for further information). Otherwise, carefully observe and record signs of chronic complications, such as retinopathy, cardiovascular disease, peripheral vascular disease, nephropathy, and neuropathies. Because diabetes mellitus causes such widespread effects, your review of all body systems provides key assessment information. Keep in mind that these effects may occur even in a patient unaware of his disease. Be sure to assess for the following:

Eye changes in the diabetic patient (diabetic retinopathy) primarily result from microvascular retinal changes. Within 10 years of onset, half of all diabetic patients have some retinopathy—and diabetes remains the leading cause of blindness between ages 20 and 65. Diabetic patients also have an increased risk of cataract formation from prolonged hyperglycemia.

Typical early eye changes include retinal microaneurysm, followed by microinfarction and exudate formation. These may progress to

Continued on page 100

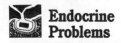
Pancreatic Disorders

Diabetes mellitus—*continued*

proliferative retinopathy, a serious condition characterized by retinal neovascularization (new blood vessel formation). Retinal detachment and vitreous hemorrhage may result (see *Staging diabetic retinopathy*).

Early retinal changes don't cause signs or symptoms, but they may be detected on eye examination. If your patient has known diabetes, advise him to have yearly eye examinations and routine blood pressure checks (hypertension's associated with an increased retinopathy incidence and progression rate).

Vascular changes may be microvascular and/or macrovascular. The patient may develop microvascular changes characterized by a thickened, damaged capillary basement membrane. These changes seem related to uncontrolled diabetes mellitus. Clinical effects of microvascular changes include retinopathy, nephropathy, and skin changes (see below). Macrovascular changes most commonly involve atherosclerosis—diabetic patients have an increased risk for atherosclerosis, develop it at an earlier age, and have more severe, extensive, and rapidly progressive disease than do nondiabetics. The diabetic patient also has an increased risk for lipid disorders, particularly hyperlipoproteinemia. And he's more likely to have hypertension, which contributes to atherosclerosis and other disorders.

Carefully assess the patient's peripheral pulses and blood pressure (in all positions). Remember that large-vessel atherosclerosis can compromise tissue oxygenation, contributing to coronary artery disease, renal stenosis, peripheral vascular disease, and cerebrovascular disease (diabetic patients may account for up to 75% of cerebrovascular accidents).

Renal changes (nephropathies) result from microvascular changes. These may include glomerular lesions, arteriosclerosis of the renal arteries or afferent or efferent arterioles, and tubular lesions. Such changes may progressively impair renal function. Look for proteinuria, an early sign of a glomerular lesion. Oliguria and increased serum creatinine and blood urea nitrogen levels may indicate renal insufficiency, which can progress to renal failure. (About 25% of Americans treated for end-stage renal disease have diabetes mellitus.)

Neurologic changes (neuropathies) may take place in the peripheral nerves, autonomic nervous system, or central nervous system, causing widely varying signs and symptoms. Peripheral neuropathies may affect both sensory and motor function (with sensory fibers usually affected first); autonomic nervous system neuropathies may cause gastric motility changes, incontinence, or impotence. Such neuropathies may stem from metabolic changes leading to sorbitol accumulation in nerve cells and in fluid shifts followed by cellular swelling, rupture, and destruction. Neuropathies may also disrupt myelin synthesis. Some neuropathies may result from vitamin deficiencies. Peripheral neuropathies, such as alcoholic neuropathy, may worsen diabetic neuropathy.

Skin changes, especially on the legs and feet, result from neuropathies and from microvascular and macrovascular changes. Examine the patient's skin closely, particularly on his legs and feet.

Continued on page 102

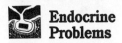
Pancreatic Disorders

Staging diabetic retinopathy

Retinopathy, a major diabetic complication and the most common cause of new blindness, may appear as an initial sign of the underlying disease or can develop many years after other diabetic signs and symptoms occur. Retinopathy chiefly involves retinal capillaries. Eventually, capillary walls weaken and develop microaneurysms. If these hemorrhage into retinal tissue, they may cause blindness from exudation into the macular region. Although retinopathy takes a variable course, the doctor will use a rough staging scheme for diagnostic purposes. The eyegrounds illustrated below show retinopathy stages as they would appear through an ophthalmoscope. Treatment of retinopathy varies with the disorder's severity.

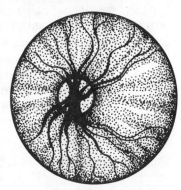

Normal retina
Pinkish orange fundus, with the optic disk located toward one side; blood vessels extending outward from the optic disk along the fundal borders

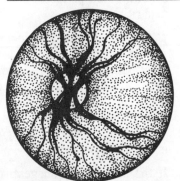

Stage I
Microaneurysms, with retinal vein distention

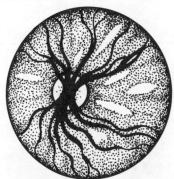

Stage II
Stage I findings plus deep retinal punctate hemorrhages and waxy exudates

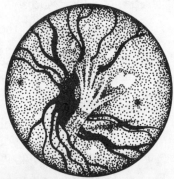

Stage III
Stage II findings plus superficial retinal images, dilatation of existing capillary networks, neovascularization, preretinal hemorrhages, and retinal surface fibrosis

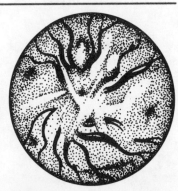

Stage IV
Stage III findings plus vitreous hemorrhages and proliferating retinopathy with its sequelae—rubeosis iridis diabetica, retinal detachment, secondary glaucoma, and useful vision loss

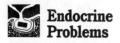
Pancreatic Disorders

Diabetes mellitus—*continued*

Look for lesions and infections that may have developed in hypertrophied skin, ingrown toenails, corns, and calluses. Check for gangrene (considerably more common in diabetic patients than in nondiabetics). Gangrene may stem from minor trauma or an undetected infection caused by sensory nerve function loss and subsequent anesthesia. Gangrene may be dry (not involving infection) or wet (associated with infection). Report signs of gangrene immediately—the patient may require amputation of the affected leg or foot. Also check for a neurotrophic ulcer, an insensitive lesion typically developing under corns and calluses; such an ulcer may progress to infection with bone involvement. Other abnormal skin lesions include reddish brown papular spots (diabetic dermopathy), which may progress to crusts and scar tissue; and necrobiosis lipoidica diabeticorum, an ulcerating, necrotic process that proves hard to control. Document your findings, and stress to the patient the need for proper foot care. (Some authorities estimate that proper foot care alone could reduce the need for amputations by up to 75%.)

Other changes include an increased risk for and susceptibility to infection. Common infections your patient may develop include *Candida* and *Staphylococcus* skin infections, vaginitis, and acute pyelonephritis.

Diagnostic studies. The doctor diagnoses diabetes mellitus from the patient's blood glucose levels. Initially, he'll probably order a fasting blood glucose level—the preferred screening test. A fasting blood glucose level of 140 mg/dl or greater on at least two occasions confirms diabetes mellitus. The American Diabetes Association (ADA) also recommends this diagnosis if the patient has a random blood glucose level of 200 mg/dl or greater as well as classic diabetes signs and symptoms.

If the patient has suggestive signs and symptoms and a fasting blood glucose level below 140 mg/dl, the doctor may order an oral glucose tolerance test to determine the insulin response to a glucose challenge. A glucose level of 200 mg/dl or greater in the 2-hour sample and in one other sample taken up to 2 hours after administration of a 75-g glucose load confirms the diagnosis.

For a pregnant patient, the doctor will use another method to establish a diagnosis. For a woman 24 to 28 weeks pregnant, he'll probably give a 100-g glucose load (as the ADA recommends). Then he'll diagnose diabetes mellitus if two samples equal or exceed these values:
- fasting—105 mg/dl
- 1-hour sample—190 mg/dl
- 2-hour sample—165 mg/dl
- 3-hour sample—145 mg/dl.

For a child, the doctor may confirm diabetes mellitus from a random blood glucose level of 200 mg/dl or greater in addition to classic diabetes signs and symptoms. He may also diagnose diabetes mellitus from fasting blood glucose levels of 140 mg/dl or greater on at least two occasions in addition to two oral glucose tolerance test results of 200 mg/dl or greater in the 2-hour sample and in one other sample taken up to 2 hours later.

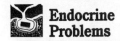
Pancreatic Disorders

Because undetected diabetes can have devastating consequences, the ADA recommends laboratory screening for the following groups:
- adults over age 40
- obese individuals
- pregnant women during weeks 24 to 28 of gestation
- women with a history of obstetric complications or gestational diabetes
- women who've delivered a baby weighing over 9 lb (4 kg)
- patients with impaired glucose tolerance
- patients with reactive hypoglycemia.

Once the doctor diagnoses diabetes mellitus, he may order ongoing urine or blood glucose testing to evaluate the patient's glucose status and his response to therapy.

Planning
Before determining your nursing care plan, develop the nursing diagnosis by identifying your patient's problem or potential problem, then relating it to its cause. Possible nursing diagnoses for a patient with diabetes mellitus include:
- knowledge deficit; related to newly diagnosed disease
- skin integrity, impairment of (potential for); related to diabetic complications
- family dynamics, alteration in; related to newly diagnosed disease
- coping, ineffective individual; related to chronic disease
- anxiety; related to daily insulin injections
- fluid volume, alteration in (deficit); related to diabetes
- noncompliance; related to inadequate health teaching.

The sample care plan on page 104 shows expected outcomes, nursing interventions, and discharge planning for one nursing diagnosis listed above. However, you'll want to tailor each care plan to the patient's needs.

Intervention
Treatment goals for the diabetic patient include:
- normalizing carbohydrate, fat, and protein metabolism
- preventing long-term complications
- ensuring normal psychosocial adaptation
- avoiding hypoglycemia and other treatment complications.

To achieve these goals, expect the doctor to use measures involving diet, insulin, sulfonylureas, exercise, glucose monitoring, and self-care techniques.

In all diabetes forms, the patient has an imbalance between available endogenous insulin and the amount his target tissues need to maintain normal metabolism. Thus, the treatment measures you implement aim to equalize the patient's insulin supply and demand. In Type II diabetic patients (about 80% of whom are obese and insulin-resistant), insulin demand increases as weight increases. Expect the doctor to order a low-calorie diet to help decrease insulin demand by reducing body weight. He may also order an exercise program, sulfonylurea drugs (which stimulate endogenous insulin secretion), or insulin therapy. For the Type I diabetic patient, the doctor will order dietary measures, exercise, and insulin therapy. If the patient develops severe insulin resistance, the doctor may also order sulfonylureas.

Continued on page 104

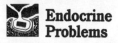
Pancreatic Disorders

Sample nursing care plan: Diabetes mellitus

Nursing diagnosis	Expected outcomes
Knowledge deficit; related to newly diagnosed disease	The patient will show that he understands: • the disease process and potential complications. • how to self-administer insulin or sulfonylureas, if indicated. • how to test his urine or blood glucose at home. • what guidelines to follow if he has hypoglycemia, hyperglycemia, or another illness. • proper hygiene, including skin, foot, and dental care. • prescribed dietary, exercise, and activity regimens.
Nursing interventions • Reinforce the need for complying with insulin or oral hypoglycemic therapy; make sure patient understands how to self-administer these drugs and recognize their adverse effects. • Discuss appropriate methods for monitoring glucose levels, such as urine or blood testing. • Discuss the need for complying with prescribed dietary, exercise, and activity regimens to maintain blood glucose control. • Make sure patient knows warning signs of hypoglycemia and hyperglycemia and appropriate treatment for each disorder. • Reinforce appropriate sick-day guidelines. • Discuss personal hygiene guidelines for skin, foot, and dental care. • Discuss methods patient can use to help prevent complications.	**Discharge planning** • Reinforce patient and family instructions. • If indicated, have patient and/or family members demonstrate insulin administration methods and glucose monitoring techniques. • Advise patient when to seek medical care. • Arrange for follow-up care if indicated. • Advise patient and family about support groups, such as the American Diabetes Association. If possible, arrange for a local group contact. • Stress the importance of regular medical care and compliance with therapy. • Arrange for a dietitian to visit with patient.

Diabetes mellitus—*continued*

Diet. Doctors regard diet as the cornerstone of diabetes care because it directly controls the body's major glucose source. Your patient's food intake must be carefully controlled to prevent widely fluctuating blood glucose levels. If he's taking insulin or sulfonylureas, he'll have to adhere to his diet even more carefully to avoid hypoglycemia.

Your patient's nutritional requirements closely resemble those of a nondiabetic: a well-balanced diet containing all the necessary nutrients. However, to avoid wide blood glucose variations, the diabetic patient needs to closely regulate his carbohydrate, protein, and fat intake. Currently, the ADA recommends that carbohydrates make up about 50% to 60% of a diabetic patient's daily intake; protein, about 10% to 15%; and fat, the remaining 30% to 35%. (The relatively low fat content may help reduce the risk of cardiovascular disease.) The Joslin Clinic's diabetic diet, an alternative regimen, recommends 40% carbohydrates, 20% protein, and 40% fat.

Discuss dietary fiber's benefits with your patient. A high fiber intake seems to improve blood glucose control, perhaps by delaying gastric emptying and slowing carbohydrate digestion and absorption. Unfortunately, the patient must consume 10 to 15 g of fiber daily for maximum benefits—not practical in most cases. Tell him, however, that he can obtain some benefit by eating such high-fiber foods as bran cereals, fresh fruits and vegetables, and legumes.

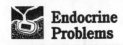
Pancreatic Disorders

Using the glycemic index to categorize foods

To improve the diabetic diet, several diabetes associations recommend that patients reduce dietary fat and substitute more foods from the carbohydrate group to make up the difference in calories. However, this requirement may pose a problem to the diabetic patient who needs to choose carbohydrates that will not cause rapid fluctuations in postprandial blood glucose levels.

Consequently, investigators now try to categorize carbohydrates according to the blood glucose level each produces after ingestion. They assign a rating, called the glycemic index, to each food. Foods with a low index don't cause rapid serum glucose increases, while those with a higher glycemic index do.

Although still experimental, the index could help patients select those carbohydrates that might minimize increases in blood glucose levels and help them adapt their diets to any ethnic or personal food preferences. Most studies tested 50 g of each carbohydrate, comparing its effect with the same quantity of white bread. (White bread was used as a standard and given a rating of 100.)

Although more testing is needed, early tests have yielded surprising results. For example, researchers found that grinding rice enhanced its glycemic effect. Pasta caused a smaller rise in postprandial blood glucose levels than bread, although both foods have a similar nutrient composition. Legumes also produced a decreased fluctuation.

For more information on using the glycemic index, consult a dietitian.

Make sure you discuss concentrated sweets (foods high in simple sugars) with the patient. Traditional diabetic diets forbid such foods as ice cream, soft drinks, cookies, candies, and pastries; researchers theorized that the body absorbs these concentrated sweets much more quickly than complex carbohydrates, with a resulting rapid blood glucose rise. However, recent studies that categorize foods according to their glycemic index (the blood glucose level after their ingestion) show that this may not be the case (see *Using the glycemic index to categorize foods*). Baked potatoes, for instance, have a higher glycemic index than ice cream. Findings such as these challenge researchers to investigate traditional diabetic diets more closely. However, don't let your patient abandon caution regarding concentrated sweets. For now, encourage him to avoid them.

Arrange for a dietitian to teach your patient how to plan his meals. Reinforce the teaching as necessary, and make sure the patient understands that meal timing proves as important as food types and amounts. Teach him to space meals (including snacks, if ordered) evenly throughout the day. The dietitian may recommend the food exchange system. This widely used method, based on the carbohydrate, fat, and protein content of six basic food groups, allows greater flexibility in meal planning. Exchange groups include milk products, vegetables, fruits, breads, meats, and fats.

Teach the patient how to adjust his diet when he engages in extra activity or exercise (see *How exercise affects the diabetic patient*, page 110). If he eats many meals out, have the dietitian show him how to select a restaurant meal that fits his diet plan; if appropriate, tell him how he can obtain nutrient composition lists from fast-food restaurants. With an overweight patient, implement weight-reduction measures, as ordered, and explain the reduced-calorie diet. Suggest a support group, such as Weight Watchers or Overeaters Anonymous, if necessary.

Insulin therapy. Only about 15% to 25% of diabetic patients require insulin therapy. These patients include:
- Type I diabetics
- Type II diabetics with hyperglycemia that's unresponsive to proper diet and oral sulfonylureas
- Type II diabetics during short periods of acute stress (for example, acute illness or surgery), when metabolic homeostasis deteriorates and blood glucose levels increase transiently.

Daily insulin therapy corrects the Type I diabetic patient's absolute insulin deficiency, corrects the relative insulin deficiency of the Type II diabetic patient unresponsive to diet and sulfonylureas, and corrects the increased insulin requirements of the Type II diabetic patient undergoing acute stress.

Insulin therapy may be prescribed singularly or in combination— the type or types used depend on the patient's hyperglycemia pattern (see *Comparing insulin types*, page 106). Such therapy aims to alleviate hyperglycemia while avoiding hypoglycemia. The doctor may prescribe a daily intermediate-acting insulin injection for one patient and a mixture of rapid-acting insulin (to control morning hyperglycemia) and intermediate-acting insulin (to control later

Continued on page 106

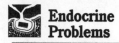
Pancreatic Disorders

Diabetes mellitus—*continued*

hyperglycemia) for another patient. Or, instead of daily injections, he may prescribe insulin on a split or mixed schedule, or continuous administration through an insulin pump (see *Insulin pumps*). To meet each patient's individual needs, effective insulin therapy must be determined by trial and error.

The doctor will consider insulin purity when developing the patient's insulin regimen. The purer the insulin, the less marked its antigenic effect. Pure pork and human insulins, for example, cause less antigenicity (and hence less insulin allergy, less insulin resistance, and less lipotrophy) than beef or beef/pork insulins. However, these purer insulins also cost more. Diabetic patients who benefit most from purified human or pork insulins include:
• Type II diabetics using insulin intermittently or for the first time
• newly diagnosed Type I diabetics
• patients with gestational diabetes or pregnant patients with previously diagnosed diabetes
• diabetics not well controlled with standard insulins
• diabetics with insulin allergy
• diabetics with severe insulin resistance.

Teach your patient how to draw up and administer his own insulin. If he needs to mix insulin types, make sure he understands the proper techniques. Stress the need for rotating injection sites, and provide him with a site rotation chart. Because the absorption rate differs at each site, most doctors recommend that the patient rotate sites within a specific area, such as the abdomen.

Comparing insulin types

SHORT-ACTING

Onset of action: 30 minutes to 1 hour
Duration: 5 to 16 hours

Standard
Regular Iletin I
Sources: Pork and beef
Concentration: U-40, U-100

Regular Insulin
Source: Pork
Concentration: U-100

Semilente Iletin
Sources: Pork and beef
Concentration: U-40, U-100

Semilente
Source: Beef
Concentration: U-100

Purified
Regular Iletin II
Source: Pork or beef
Concentration: U-100

Regular Purified
Source: Pork
Concentration: U-100

Velosulin
Source: Pork
Concentration: U-100

Humulin R
Source: Human
Concentration: U-100

Novolin R
Source: Human
Concentration: U-100

INTERMEDIATE-ACTING

Onset of action: 1 to 2 hours
Duration: 16 to 28 hours

Standard
NPH Iletin I
Sources: Pork and beef
Concentration U-40, U-100

Lente Iletin I
Sources: Pork and beef
Concentration: U-40, U-100

NPH Insulin
Source: Beef
Concentration: U-100

Lente
Source: Beef
Concentration: U-100

Purified
NPH Iletin II
Source: Pork or beef
Concentration: U-100

Lente Iletin II
Source: Pork or beef
Concentration: U-40, U-100

NPH Purified
Source: Pork
Concentration: U-100

Lente Purified
Source: Pork
Concentration: U-100

Insulatard NPH
Source: Pork
Concentration: U-100

Mixtard
Source: Pork
Concentration: U-100

Humulin N
Source: Human
Concentration: U-100

Novolin N
Source: Human
Concentration: U-100

Novolin L
Source: Human
Concentration: U-100

LONG-ACTING

Onset of action: 3 to 8 hours
Duration: 36 hours or more

Standard
Ultralente Iletin I
Sources: Pork and beef
Concentration: U-40, U-100

PZI Iletin I
Sources: Pork and beef
Concentration: U-40, U-100

Ultralente
Source: Beef
Concentration: U-100

Purified
PZI Iletin II
Source: Pork or beef
Concentration: U-100

Ultralente Purified
Source: Beef
Concentration: U-100

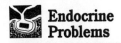
Pancreatic Disorders

Insulin pumps

For a patient who needs long-term insulin therapy, an insulin pump offers several advantages over such conventional insulin delivery methods as standard injection and jet injection.

Insulin pumps work on either a closed-loop or an open-loop system. The self-contained closed-loop system both detects and responds to changing blood glucose levels (for this reason, it's sometimes called an artificial beta cell).

The Biostator Glucose Controller, the only currently available closed-loop system, contains a glucose sensor, a programmable computer, a power supply, a pump, and an insulin reservoir. The computer triggers continuous insulin delivery in appropriate amounts from the reservoir. This model does have a drawback—it's used only in hospitals because of its large size and because it withdraws blood and infuses insulin I.V. A smaller version currently under development would be implanted under the patient's skin.

The open-loop pump infuses insulin but can't respond to blood glucose changes. Also called a Continuous Subcutaneous Insulin Infuser, the pump delivers insulin in small (basal) doses every few minutes and in large (bolus) doses that the patient sets manually. The system consists of a reservoir containing regular insulin, a small pump, an infusion rate selector allowing insulin release adjustments, a battery, and a plastic catheter with an attached needle leading from the syringe to the subcutaneous injection site. The patient can fasten the pump to his belt or other waist-level clothing (see illustration below).

The infusion rate selector automatically releases about half the total daily insulin requirement. The patient releases the remainder in bolus amounts before meals and snacks. The patient must change the syringe daily and must change the needle, catheter, and injection site every other day.

Patients who benefit most from an insulin pump include:
• those with widely fluctuating blood glucose levels despite optimal insulin and dietary regimens
• those whose job or life-style prevents regular meals
• pregnant women.

The doctor probably won't order an insulin pump for the following patients:
• those who won't comply with standard dietary, insulin, and self-monitoring regimens
• those who miss scheduled medical appointments
• those who can't recognize hypoglycemia symptoms
• those with diabetic complications, such as advanced renal disease, proliferative retinopathy, or severe autonomic neuropathy.

Despite recent advances that have rendered insulin pumps smaller and more programmable, the devices do have potential drawbacks. These include infection at injection sites, catheter clogging, and insulin loss from a loose reservoir-catheter connection.

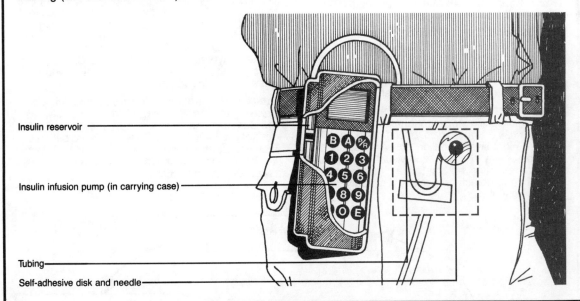

Insulin reservoir

Insulin infusion pump (in carrying case)

Tubing

Self-adhesive disk and needle

Complications of insulin therapy include hypoglycemia, the Somogyi phenomenon (see *Recognizing the Somogyi phenomenon*, page 108), insulin lipodystrophy (subcutaneous tissue hypertrophy or atrophy, usually caused by continuously using the same injection site), insulin allergy, and insulin resistance.

Sulfonylurea therapy. American doctors currently prescribe six different sulfonylureas to treat Type II diabetic patients unresponsive to diet alone. Traditional sulfonylureas (first-generation hypogly-

Continued on page 108

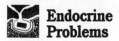
Pancreatic Disorders

Diabetes mellitus—*continued*

cemic agents) include tolbutamide, tolazamide, acetohexamide, and chlorpropamide. Newer sulfonylureas (second-generation hypoglycemic agents) include glipizide and glyburide. Sulfonylureas initially regulate blood glucose levels by increasing beta cell insulin secretion. This effect diminishes after several months, but the drugs also have a second, more important effect—they decrease cellular insulin resistance, enhancing blood glucose regulation. Some doctors prescribe sulfonylureas for Type I diabetic patients with severe insulin resistance resulting from acquired insulin antigenicity, but this use remains controversial.

Diabetic patients who benefit most from sulfonylurea therapy include:
• those who developed diabetes after age 40
• those who've had diabetes for less than 5 years

Recognizing the Somogyi phenomenon

The Somogyi phenomenon—insulin rebound syndrome—can occur when your patient receives too much insulin. Normally, you'd expect overinsulinization to cause *hypoglycemia*. But when the Somogyi phenomenon kicks in, the body's normal defense mechanisms overreact to hypoglycemia and cause abundant secretion of glucocorticoids, epinephrine, glucagon, and growth hormone. Because these hormones counter insulin's action, *hyperglycemia* sets in, suggesting a need for *more* insulin. Of course, administering more insulin only worsens the problem, causing even more severe hypoglycemia and rebound hyperglycemia (see flowchart below). At this point, the patient needs *less* insulin.

Assessment. You can't correct this problem unless you recognize it—and recognition can be tricky. Rule out dietary deviations as the cause of poor control, and consider that patients under unusual stress (as with pregnancy or surgery) more greatly risk the Somogyi phenomenon.

First, check for classic hypoglycemia signs and symptoms—sweating, warmth, restlessness, lightheadedness, tremors, palpitations, weakness, hunger, night sweats, pallor, drowsiness, insomnia, personality changes, and visual disturbances. Remember, however, that these changes may be too subtle to detect—especially if hypoglycemia occurs only at night.

Characteristic temperature and blood pressure changes also suggest the Somogyi phenomenon. During a hypoglycemic episode, body temperature and diastolic pressure typically drop slightly while systolic pressure increases slightly.

Also evaluate urine or blood glucose trends for several negative results followed by several positive results. To confirm the pattern, monitor blood glucose levels every few hours. Glucose testing proves crucial for detecting this phenomenon because signs and symptoms of recurring hypoglycemia may be subtle enough to escape detection. Because hypoglycemia commonly occurs at night, monitor blood glucose levels throughout the night as well. Your patient will probably have hypoglycemia for a day, then hyperglycemia for one or more days. However, his glucose level may fluctuate between hyperglycemia and hypoglycemia within a single day; if you test at only one time you may get a misleading result.

Intervention. Treatment involves cautiously *decreasing* the insulin dose. If the patient truly has the Somogyi phenomenon, he'll show improved control with less insulin. Type I diabetic patients may need a reduction of only a few units of insulin. Type II diabetic patients on insulin may need reductions of up to 30%.

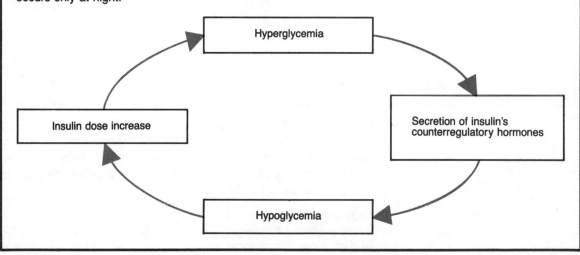

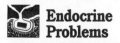
Pancreatic Disorders

Sulfonylureas

Acetohexamide (Dymelor)
Duration of action: 12 to 18 hours

Chlorpropamide (Diabinese)
Duration of action: 60 hours

Glipizide (Glucotrol)
Duration of action: up to 24 hours

Glyburide (DiaBeta, Micronase)
Duration of action: up to 24 hours

Tolazamide (Tolinase)
Duration of action: 12 to 24 hours

Tolbutamide (Orinase)
Duration of action: 6 to 12 hours

Phenformin: Available for a select few

Phenformin (formerly DBI-TD), a biguanide oral hypoglycemic agent, was removed from the United States market in 1977, when researchers linked it with an unacceptably high risk of lactic acidosis. However, a few patients still need phenformin to control diabetes mellitus. Recognizing this, the Food and Drug Administration (FDA) makes the drug available through an Investigational New Drug application, which a prescribing doctor must file with the FDA.

According to the FDA, phenformin may be used only in nonketotic diabetic patients who meet *all* these criteria:
• elevated blood glucose levels
• hyperglycemia signs and symptoms
• signs and symptoms that persist despite dietary measures or sulfonylurea therapy (or hypersensitivity to sulfonylureas)
• responsiveness to phenformin
• no underlying risk factors contraindicating phenformin use
• hypoglycemia risk from insulin, threatening the patient's job or posing a hazard to him or others
• disability that bars insulin self-administration, if the patient has no practical way to get help.

If your patient's taking phenformin, advise him to avoid alcoholic beverages. Make sure he recognizes the signs and symptoms that herald lactic acidosis (nausea, vomiting, hyperventilation, malaise, and abdominal pain). If any of these occur, he should stop taking the drug and notify his doctor immediately.

• those with normal or above-normal body weight
• those needing less than 40 units of insulin to achieve good control.

Diabetic patients who shouldn't receive these agents include:
• pregnant or breast-feeding women (effects on the fetus and newborn haven't been determined)
• those experiencing stressful concurrent conditions or illnesses, who have variable but increased insulin requirements
• those with allergies to sulfa agents.

If your patient's taking a sulfonylurea, teach him about the particular agent. Stress that the drug doesn't replace dietary measures but works *with* them to help improve blood glucose control. Review the drug's potential adverse effects, and tell the patient to report them to his doctor if they occur. Make sure he and his family understand how to recognize hypoglycemia signs and symptoms and how to intervene appropriately if they occur. Advise the patient to take the drug only as ordered and never to alter the frequency or dose without consulting his doctor. In particular, tell him never to discontinue the drug without medical advice because uncontrolled hyperglycemia might result. Review guidelines for alcohol use—sulfonylureas may cause alcohol intolerance and hypoglycemia.

Exercise. This important but sometimes neglected treatment measure effectively lowers blood glucose levels by enhancing cellular glucose uptake without necessitating additional insulin. However, it's effective only when performed consistently.

The doctor will tailor the exercise plan to the patient's physical condition, medical status, and risk for complications. If necessary, suggest a consultation with a physical therapist, who can help plan an appropriate program.

Help the patient choose an *aerobic* exercise, such as walking, running, cycling, or swimming. Aerobic exercises use glucose as fuel, thus decreasing blood glucose levels. They also have cardiovascular benefits—important for the diabetic patient who risks cardiovascular disease. Tell the patient to avoid *anaerobic* exercises, such as weight lifting or push-ups. These don't use glucose as fuel and can *increase* blood glucose levels as the body reacts to exercise-induced stress. Anaerobic exercises also cause rapid heart rate and blood pressure increases—potentially dangerous for any patient prone to cardiovascular disease.

Tell your patient to exercise at least three times a week on alternate days, with each session lasting between 45 and 60 minutes. Advise him to include the following phases in his exercise program to avoid complications:
• *Warm-up.* This phase, which consists of 5 to 10 minutes of slow exercise, increases the heart rate safely and stretches muscles gradually.
• *Conditioning.* The exercise program's main component, this phase should last 25 to 30 minutes. The body burns glucose as the patient strives to reach his target heart rate. If feasible, suggest that the patient have a stress electrocardiogram to determine his target heart rate. If this isn't possible, have him determine his target rate by subtracting his age from 220 and multiplying the result by 0.7.

Continued on page 111

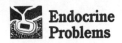

Pancreatic Disorders

How exercise affects the diabetic patient

To get a picture of the physiologic effects of exercise, think of the body as the energy supplier, the circulatory system as the energy pipeline, and the muscle as the energy user. Here—as with other bodily functions—the law of supply and demand prevails, and that means the energy in the pipeline must remain even at all times. As you'd expect, that's where the diabetic patient runs into trouble. To understand why, first consider the physiologic effects of exercise on a nondiabetic person.

A resting muscle gets by on the energy it draws from free fatty acids (FFAs). But once that muscle starts exercising, it needs an additional energy source. At first, intramuscular glycogen, adenosine triphosphate, and creatinine supply the extra energy. But soon even that's not enough, and the muscle starts drawing on blood glucose.

After just 10 minutes of exercise, the muscle's glucose uptake can be 15 times higher than basal value; after 60 minutes, more than 35 times higher. At that point, FFAs provide only about 40% of the muscle's energy, with the rest coming from blood glucose and glycogen. After 3 or 4 hours of activity, the muscle reverts to FFAs as its primary energy source—like getting a second wind. Even so, it continues using more blood glucose than it did before it started exercising.

The hormonal system keeps blood glucose on an even keel by regulating glucose and FFA metabolism. The insulin level drops, so hepatic output and lipolysis improve; catecholamine, cortisol, glucagon, and growth hormone levels increase, which also stimulates hepatic output and lipolysis. As a result, the blood glucose level doesn't climb

or drop. Increased glucose use balances increased glucose production, so glucose levels in the "pipeline" stay even.

For a person with diabetes, however, increased glucagon, cortisol, and growth hormone levels can greatly exceed what's needed, so he produces too much glucose. His plasma catecholamines can increase twofold or threefold, increasing not just glucose production but pulse rate and blood pressure as well. His injected insulin can be mobilized prematurely, causing his insulin level to climb rather than drop. If his insulin level's too low or just inadequate (a blood glucose level over 240 mg/dl), exercise will increase the blood glucose level. That's because his body continues to release glucose from the liver but can't move it into the exercising muscle. With everything going helter-skelter, his blood glucose can't remain on an even keel.

You can see why a diabetic patient might easily become discouraged with exercise. But he needn't be. If he undertakes the exercise when his insulin level's adequate, he might *reduce* his blood glucose level. That's because the circulating insulin both suppresses glucose formation in the liver and increases the muscles' glucose uptake.

Even after he finishes exercising, his body needs a few hours to replenish hepatic and muscle glycogen, so his blood glucose level stays low. With this prolonged blood glucose decrease, the need for exogenous insulin can be dramatically reduced, and the need for sulfonylureas can be eliminated. But the patient needs the right exercise program to begin with, and he must perform it regularly. If he stops, the benefits stop.

EXERCISE				DIETARY ADJUSTMENTS*	
Intensity	Cal/hour	Examples	Duration	15 to 30 minutes before exercise	During exercise
Mild	50 to 199	Standing Strolling (1 mph) Light housework	Less than 30 minutes	None	None
			More than 30 minutes	None	None
Moderate	200 to 299	Walking (2 mph) Vacuuming Bowling Playing golf	Less than 30 minutes	None	None
			More than 30 minutes	None	5 g simple carbohydrate every 30 minutes
Marked	300 to 399	Jogging (3 to 4 mph) Swimming Scrubbing floors	Less than 30 minutes	15 to 20 g complex carbohydrate, plus protein	None
			More than 30 minutes	15 to 20 g complex carbohydrate, plus protein	10 g simple carbohydrate every 30 minutes
Vigorous	Over 400	Jogging (5 mph) Skiing Playing tennis	Less than 30 minutes	30 to 40 g complex carbohydrate, plus protein	None
			More than 30 minutes	30 to 40 g complex carbohydrate, plus protein	10 to 20 g simple carbohydrate every 30 minutes

*These adjustments represent guidelines; specific adjustments should be based on the results of individual glucose monitoring.

Pancreatic Disorders

Diabetes mellitus: Patient teaching tips

Patient and family teaching prove crucial to successful diabetes mellitus management. Include these topics in your teaching program:
- disease definition
- diet therapy and nutrition
- exercise
- insulin or sulfonylurea therapy
- glucose-monitoring techniques
- hypoglycemia prevention and treatment
- skin hygiene and foot care
- sick-day guidelines
- psychological adjustment.

Diabetes mellitus—*continued*

For example, the target heart rate for a patient age 40 would be 126 (220 − 40 = 175 × 0.7).
- *Cool-down.* In this final phase, which lasts about 15 minutes, the patient performs exercises designed to gradually reduce his heart rate to normal.

Teach your patient how to take his pulse, and tell him to do so before and after he exercises as well as during the conditioning phase. Advise him never to exceed his target heart rate, because this increases the risk of complications. Make sure you review with the patient how exercise affects blood glucose levels and the safety guidelines he should follow.

Glucose monitoring. Because blood glucose changes may cause misleading signs and symptoms—or none at all—the diabetic patient must measure his glucose level, perhaps several times a day.

Urine testing. Depending on the patient's disease, life-style, physical limitations, and visual acuity, the doctor may order any of various urine testing kits. Teach the patient how to use the prescribed equipment, and tell him to record his glycosuria reading as a percentage rather than in plus marks (for example, + or + +). Plus marks don't correlate with the same percentages on all urine tests and may cause interpretation errors. If the patient has a renal threshold of 180 mg/dl or more, explain that negative urine test results mask significant hyperglycemia; suggest blood glucose monitoring as an alternative. As ordered, tell the patient what to do if his urine tests abnormally.

Urine testing can detect *ketone bodies*—particularly important for the ketosis-prone diabetic patient. Encourage urine ketone testing for all Type I diabetics (routine daily testing) and for any diabetic patient who feels ill.

Teach the patient how to test his urine for ketone bodies. Keep in mind that urine ketone testing also benefits the Type I diabetic patient on blood glucose self-monitoring (see below).

Despite its convenience, urine testing has several disadvantages:
- Tests don't always reflect blood glucose levels accurately (some patients with high blood glucose levels may have negative urine test results; some patients with low blood glucose levels may have positive urine test results).
- The renal threshold for glucose spillage into urine increases with the patient's age, making glycosuria harder to detect.
- A time lag separates hyperglycemia and urine glucose appearance.
- Tests can't reveal hypoglycemia.

Blood glucose self-monitoring. An increasing number of diabetic patients use this self-monitoring technique to avoid urine testing's drawbacks. The technique's especially useful for those on a tight-control regimen that aims to maintain blood glucose levels as close to normal as possible while avoiding hypoglycemia. It allows the patient to determine his metabolic status at a glance, permitting more immediate feedback about adjustments or noncompliance with his diet or insulin regimen.

Continued on page 113

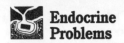
Pancreatic Disorders

Glucose monitoring techniques

Blood or urine glucose testing monitors glucose levels in the patient with diabetes mellitus. Blood glucose tests, considered more reliable than urine tests, include reagent strips, glucose meters, and glycohemoglobin tests.

Reagent strips include the Chemstrip bG and Visidex. To use a reagent strip, the patient draws a blood droplet—usually by fingertip puncture with a manual device such as the Monolet lancet or a mechanical device such as the Autolet, the Hemalet, the Penlet, or the Monojector. Tell the patient to follow the package instructions carefully.

The glucose meter, such as the Glucometer II, Glucoscan II, or Accu-Chek bG, offers more precise blood glucose measurement than the patient can get with visual testing. However, it's a more expensive method. Before using a meter, the patient may need to complete its calibration and control procedures. Calibration checks only the meter's accuracy. The control procedure checks the accuracy of the entire system: the meter, reagent strips, and the user's technique (timing, flushing, and strip blotting). Instruct the patient to follow the manufacturer's instructions.

The glycohemoglobin test (also called the glycosylated hemoglobin or hemoglobin A_{1c} test) reveals the patient's blood glucose level over the previous 3 months. By eliminating short-term variations, it helps evaluate the long-term effectiveness of diabetes therapy. Here's how the test works:

Hemoglobin contains hemoglobin A (90% to 95%) and three variants—hemoglobin A_{1a}, A_{1b}, and A_{1c}. These factors, collectively called glycohemoglobin or glycosylated hemoglobin, derive from a different globin chain and make up about 4% to 8% of total hemoglobin. Most diabetic patients have a larger glycohemoglobin percentage than do nondiabetics. Because glycosylation occurs at a constant rate during a red blood cell's 120-day life span, glycosylated hemoglobin levels reflect the patient's average blood glucose level during the preceding 3 months. A level that's 7.5% or lower than the normal blood glucose range shows good diabetic control; 7.6% to 8.9%, fair control; 9.0% or more, poor control.

Urine glucose tests include Clinitest tablets, reagent strips, and paper tape. These tests don't necessarily reflect blood glucose concentration. Glucose in the glomerular filtrate undergoes reabsorption until the tubules can no longer remove glucose. Normally, this occurs at about 160 to 180 mg/dl—the renal glucose threshold. But individual variations and kidney function changes can alter this level. The urine glucose level (called the urine fractional) serves as an index for assessing blood glucose control.

Clinitest tablets detect glycosuria. If your patient's using these tablets, tell him to follow these important guidelines:
• Use only freshly voided urine.
• Place 2 or 5 urine drops (or as indicated) and 10 water drops in a clean test tube, then add 1 Clinitest tablet. (*Note:* Use only fresh whole tablets that dissolve completely and always use the Clinitest dropper.)
• Don't shake the tube during the reaction.
• About 15 seconds after the reaction stops, compare urine color to the proper color chart.

Because the Clinitest depends on copper reduction of sugars (including glucose), other urine sugars can cause false-positive results. Large vitamin C doses, large aspirin doses (more than six tablets daily), and use of such drugs as sulfisoxazole, levodopa, probenecid, and isoniazid can also result in false-positive results. Cephalosporins may cause color reactions that make Clinitest results difficult to read.

Reagent strips and paper tape methods include such tests as Diastix, Keto-Diastix, Clinistix, and Tes-Tape. These tests—specific for glucose—show urine glucose—oxidase reactions. If your patient's using either type, tell him to dip the strip or paper tape quickly in and out of the urine, then hold it in the air to read it. Use of ascorbic acid, pyridium, salicylates, and levodopa can alter test results.

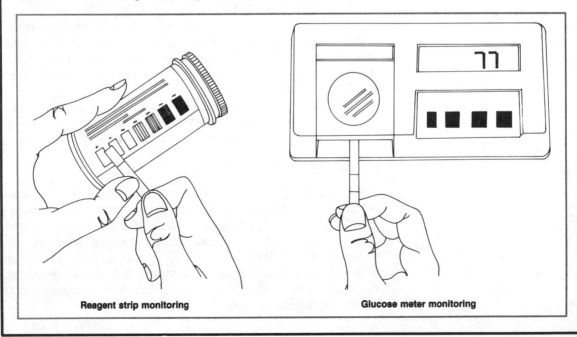

Reagent strip monitoring   **Glucose meter monitoring**

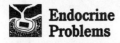
Pancreatic Disorders

Diabetes mellitus—*continued*

Other patients who may benefit from blood glucose self-monitoring include:
- brittle (unstable) diabetics, for whom hypoglycemia poses a constant danger
- diabetics contemplating pregnancy (tight blood glucose control before conception and during pregnancy greatly reduces the risk of infant mortality and hyperglycemia-related birth defects)
- diabetics using multiple daily insulin injections or an insulin pump.

Your patient can select from several types of self-monitoring equipment. Some tests use a reflectance meter, which gives a precise numerical value for blood glucose levels. Other tests (for example, Chemstrip bG and Visidex II) don't involve a meter, but indicate a blood glucose value range by visual inspection. For many patients, knowing the range suffices.

Teach your patient how to stick his finger to obtain test blood, how to apply a blood droplet to the test strip, and how to read the results (see *Glucose monitoring techniques*). Remind him that good technique and accurate timing help ensure reliable results. Instruct him to perform the test at the specified times—depending on the patient's condition, the doctor may order testing before meals, after meals, and at bedtime, or he may order a more infrequent schedule for a patient who's established stable control. Remind the patient of hypoglycemia and hyperglycemia signs and symptoms, and tell him that self-monitoring can validate subjective symptoms.

Hemoglobin A_{1c} monitoring. Monitoring of glycosylated hemoglobin (hemoglobin A_{1c})—a minor hemoglobin that results from normal hemoglobin A glycosylation—helps assess long-term diabetes control. The amount of glycosylation (glucose adherence to the hemoglobin protein) directly correlates with blood glucose levels. Because hemoglobin A_{1c} accumulates over the red blood cells' 120-day life span, levels reflect the *average* blood glucose level over several months.

Ideally, the patient's hemoglobin A_{1c} should measure no more than 1.5 times the normal level (which ranges from 3% to 6%). A high hemoglobin A_{1c} value with any blood glucose level suggests hyperglycemia over several weeks; a low value coupled with a high blood glucose level suggests recent hyperglycemia onset.

Self-care techniques. The diabetic patient can play a crucial role in preventing or minimizing diabetic complications by participating in his own care. Self-care techniques (besides compliance with diet and medication regimens) include:
- recognition, prevention, and treatment of hypoglycemia and hyperglycemia
- meticulous skin and foot care
- adherence to sick-day guidelines.

Recognition, prevention, and treatment. Because the patient's blood glucose level may change at any time, make sure he understands the signs and symptoms, prevention, and treatment of hypoglycemia and hyperglycemia. Remind him that hypoglycemia may result from too much insulin, too little food, unusually strenuous exercise, or a delayed meal. Hypoglycemia signs and symptoms include head-

Continued on page 114

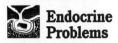
Pancreatic Disorders

Both diagnostic testing and surgery pose certain risks to the diabetic patient. Keep the following important points in mind to help prevent or minimize these risks:

Diagnostic testing. Hypoglycemia may occur when a patient taking insulin or sulfonylureas undergoes a fasting test. Check with the doctor and, as ordered, keep glucose available during the test. Or delay insulin or sulfonylurea administration, as ordered, until the patient finishes the test. If possible, schedule diagnostic tests in the early morning to minimize disruption of the patient's drug regimen.

Surgery. A physiologic and psychological stress for anyone, surgery poses added risks to the diabetic patient, including:
• decreased infection resistance
• microvascular and macrovascular complications
• impaired wound healing
• hypoglycemia or hyperglycemia. Lack of oral intake decreases available calories and may reduce insulin needs; however, hormonal responses to surgically induced stress may elevate blood glucose levels and increase insulin needs.

As with diagnostic testing, surgery should be scheduled early in the day to help minimize metabolic disruption.

If you're caring for an insulin-dependent diabetic who's scheduled for surgery, expect to administer glucose I.V. on the morning of surgery and to give an adjusted insulin dose. Postoperatively, give glucose I.V., as ordered, until the patient can take food orally. Also give insulin by subcutaneous injection in equally divided doses, or added to I.V. fluids, as ordered. Monitor the patient's blood or urine glucose level every 4 to 6 hours, as indicated.

If your patient's a non-insulin-dependent diabetic, expect to administer glucose I.V. on the morning of surgery. Postoperatively, monitor blood glucose and urine glucose and ketone levels every 4 to 6 hours. Depending on test results, give insulin, as ordered.

With any diabetic patient who's recovering from surgery, give 125
Continued

Diabetes mellitus—*continued*

ache, excessive sweating, faintness, palpitations, trembling, impaired vision, hunger, irritability, and personality changes. If the patient notices these, tell him to increase his blood glucose level by taking appropriate measures (see *Emergency hypoglycemia intervention,* page 127).

Hyperglycemia, on the other hand, may result from too little insulin, dietary noncompliance, infection, illness, or emotional distress. Signs and symptoms include increased thirst, urination, glycosuria, weakness, abdominal pain, generalized aches, deep breathing, appetite loss, nausea, and vomiting. If the patient notices these, tell him to call his doctor immediately, to take fluids without sugar if he can swallow, and to test his glucose level frequently. Teach him to help prevent these episodes by adhering to his diet, medication, exercise regimens, and sick-day guidelines.

Meticulous skin and foot care. This helps avoid problems associated with peripheral vascular disease and neuropathy. Because even a tiny skin break (particularly on the legs and feet) can eventually lead to devastating complications necessitating amputation, teach the patient to take precautions to avoid even slight trauma. Have him follow these guidelines:
• Inspect the skin daily and look for small breaks, especially between the toes and around the toenails. Closely examine each foot sole and the skin under fat folds.
• Cleanse the skin daily with soap and warm water. Check water temperature first; otherwise, neuropathy (sensation loss) may result in a bad burn. Bath water should range between 90° and 95° F. (32.2° to 35° C.).
• Always dry skin gently. To prevent tissue damage, avoid vigorous rubbing, particularly of the legs and feet.
• Apply lotion after bathing to alleviate dry skin. However, don't put lotion between the toes—this moist area promotes bacterial growth.
• Wear clean socks and underwear each day. Use only cotton items, which absorb perspiration best, and make sure they fit well. Avoid tight-fitting garments (such as girdles and tight stockings), which may impair leg and foot circulation.
• Wear leather shoes, if possible—synthetic materials trap perspiration and may lead to fungal infections and blisters. Buy shoes late in the day, when feet swell; break in new shoes gradually to avoid blisters and subsequent infection.
• Never go barefoot, and always wear socks with shoes.
• Have a podiatrist remove corns and calluses—commercial preparations may be too harsh for a diabetic patient's sensitive skin. Never use a razor blade to remove calluses, because this may cause injury leading to infection.
• Cut toenails straight across, no shorter than the toe tip. If your vision's impaired, have a family member perform this task or consult a podiatrist.
• If an injury does occur, wash the area with warm water and soap and apply a dry, sterile dressing. Don't use iodine or other harsh antiseptics, which may cause further damage. Change the dressing

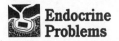
Pancreatic Disorders

to 250 g carbohydrate daily, as ordered, until he resumes his normal diet. Once he's eating normally, continue to monitor his blood glucose and urine glucose and ketone levels—he may need extra insulin from surgically induced glucose catabolism.

several times daily and inspect the area closely. If it becomes red, hot, swollen, or painful, or if you see drainage on the dressing, call the doctor at once. If the injury involves a leg, don't use the leg until the injury heals. Promote healing by elevating the leg as much as possible to increase circulation.

Adherence to sick-day guidelines. This helps balance the metabolic upsets that illness can cause. Stress, as occurs with illness, leads to release of certain hormones that increase blood glucose levels. And illness frequently alters dietary intake, causing further complications for the diabetic patient on insulin or sulfonylureas. Tell your patient to follow these guidelines when he's sick:

● Take insulin as prescribed, but call your doctor—he may adjust the dose.

● Increase your fluid intake.

● Monitor urine or blood glucose levels more frequently than usual.

● If illness reduces your dietary intake, spread half your daily carbohydrate allowance over 24 hours.

● If you can't tolerate solid foods, include dietary items with more

Continued on page 116

Pancreas and islet cell transplantation

Pancreas and islet cell transplantation, both experimental, help treat diabetes mellitus. Despite the obvious risks of rejection and infection, the procedures have produced encouraging results.

In *pancreas transplantation,* the doctor removes the pancreatic body and tail and anastomoses the splenic artery (or celiac axis) and splenic (or portal) vein to the recipient's iliac vessels (see illustrations below). This method has largely replaced pancreaticoduodenal transplantation, a more extensive procedure involving removal of the duodenum, portal vein, and an aortic patch as well as the pancreas. The simpler segmental pancreas transplantation permits organ donation from living relatives (more than half the pancreas can be removed from a normal individual without serious consequences). Most patients receiving pancreas transplants have end-stage diabetic glomerulopathy and receive a renal transplant at the same time to prevent or relieve vascular diabetic complications. Some patients without renal disease have also received these transplants.

The patient requires immunosuppressive therapy—most commonly, with cyclosporine A—to prevent organ rejection. To relieve the drug's toxic effects on the liver and kidney, the doctor may use it in combination with more conventional therapy, such as prednisone or azathioprine.

To control pancreatic secretions, the doctor may choose a drainage or suppression technique, for example, deliberate cutaneous fistula, duct ligation, ductoureterostomy, free peritoneal drainage, or pancreatic duct occlusion by synthetic polymers (such as prolamine or neoprene).

Islet cell transplantation helps restore normal serum glucose and insulin levels. The doctor transplants fetal or adult islet cell tissue (from a human donor or cadaver) into such sites as the portal vein, muscle, or spleen. The patient requires immunosuppressive therapy.

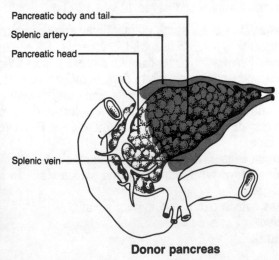

Pancreatic body and tail
Splenic artery
Pancreatic head
Splenic vein

Donor pancreas

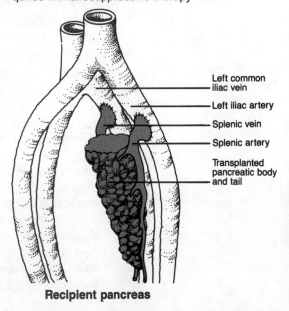

Left common iliac vein
Left iliac artery
Splenic vein
Splenic artery
Transplanted pancreatic body and tail

Recipient pancreas

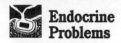
Pancreatic Disorders

Diabetes mellitus—*continued*

simple sugars than normally allowed (for example, custard, gelatin, and nondiet soft drinks).
• Return to your normal prescribed diet as soon as possible.

Emphasize the importance of taking daily insulin even if the patient changes his dietary habits. Explain that because stress raises blood glucose levels even if the patient doesn't eat, he should contact his doctor to determine whether to alter his normal insulin dose. Encourage the patient to follow common illness guidelines, such as drinking fluids, staying in bed, and taking his temperature frequently. Instruct him to increase glucose testing to every 4 hours, or as ordered, and to begin urine ketone testing. Advise him to call his doctor if testing reveals steadily increasing hyperglycemia, constant hyperglycemia above his normal pattern, or urine ketones. He should also call his doctor if he's insulin-dependent and becomes too sick to eat normally or remain active.

Tell him not to stay alone, because hyperglycemia may worsen and lead to reduced awareness and perception. A family member or friend must contact a doctor at once if the patient can't do so himself—for example, if he has difficulty breathing or if he becomes sleepy and has difficulty concentrating.

Other measures. A diabetic patient may benefit from pancreas or islet cell transplantation (see *Pancreas and islet cell transplantation,* page 115). In addition, current studies involving cyclosporine A may eventually lead to the use of this immunosuppressive to combat islet cell–destroying antibodies in early Type I diabetes mellitus.

Complications

Despite its usual chronic nature, diabetes mellitus occasionally leads to severe increases in blood glucose and/or ketone acid levels. These life-threatening complications include two major syndromes that we'll discuss below:
• diabetic ketoacidosis—glucose and ketone accumulation
• hyperglycemic hyperosmolar nonketotic coma—glucose accumulation without ketones.

These disorders may cause death rapidly unless the patient's promptly assessed and treated. (For information on hypoglycemia—another common complication—see pages 122 to 129.)

Diabetic ketoacidosis (DKA). An acute metabolic emergency characterized by significant hyperglycemia and ketonemia, DKA can rapidly lead to severe dehydration (from osmotic diuresis), metabolic acidosis (from hyperketonemia), electrolyte depletion (from osmotic diuresis), and hyperosmolarity (from hyperglycemia and dehydration). These abnormalities result directly from an absolute or relative insulin lack, which may develop over several hours or days. Possible causes of DKA include:
• infection (a common cause), which increases metabolism
• improper or inadequate insulin administration, which leads to a glucose-insulin imbalance
• emotional distress, which can cause hyperglycemia
• decreased exercise
• increased food intake.

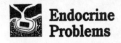
Pancreatic Disorders

Both deficient insulin relative to glucose needs and excess counterregulatory hormones contribute to DKA. Without insulin to transport glucose into cells, blood glucose levels increase. When the kidneys reach their glucose resorption threshold, some glucose spills into the urine. Hyperglycemia then initiates osmotic diuresis, drawing fluid from intracellular and interstitial spaces into the intravascular space.

Meanwhile, increased secretion of counterregulatory hormones—glucagon, epinephrine, cortisol, and growth hormone—contributes to and sustains hyperglycemia. Also, to compensate for deficient carbohydrate fuels, fat metabolism begins. However, fat doesn't burn completely to carbon dioxide, water, and energy. Instead, incomplete fat metabolism with free fatty acid release results in excess ketone bodies or ketoacids (ketonemia). Glycerol, another fat metabolism by-product, further increases the blood glucose level.

Hyperglycemia and ketonemia lead to a critical water, calorie, and electrolyte loss. Severe osmotic diuresis takes place, with loss of sodium, potassium, chloride, magnesium, and phosphate. Hemoconcentration can also develop, with decreased vascular volume. The large water loss causes polyuria. Any nausea and vomiting further contribute to fluid and electrolyte loss.

Ketosis results in metabolic acidosis with excess hydrogen ion concentration. Compensatory mechanisms attempt to correct this. The kidneys excrete ketones and increase hydrogen ion excretion by secreting ammonia. The respiratory center initiates rapid, deep respirations (Kussmaul's respirations) in an effort to blow off excess carbonic acid as water and CO_2. As these mechanisms fail, death results unless the condition's treated.

The patient with DKA appears acutely ill, with multiple signs and symptoms. Initial findings include those of untreated diabetes mellitus (polyuria, polydipsia, polyphagia, weight loss, and fatigue). As fat breakdown begins and serum ketone bodies accumulate, osmotic diuresis and dehydration worsen, and Kussmaul's respirations and acetone (fruity) breath odor occur. The patient may have facial flushing from fever, dehydration, or superficial vasodilation secondary to carbonic acid increase. Fluid loss, sodium loss, or neuropathy may lead to abdominal pain. As DKA progresses, decreasing cardiac output from volume depletion produces hypotension, with reduced vital-organ perfusion. Mental changes may range from confusion to coma.

Strongly suspect DKA if you detect these three critical signs:
• Kussmaul's respirations
• acetone breath odor
• severe dehydration.

The doctor will confirm the diagnosis from the patient's clinical condition, history, and laboratory test results. Diagnostic studies typically include a blood glucose test revealing hyperglycemia; urine and blood tests showing acetone; arterial blood gas measurements reflecting decreased pH and subnormal CO_2 levels; electrolyte imbalance; and an EKG reflecting potassium imbalance (from insulin deficiency causing intracellular potassium to enter extracellular fluid).

Continued on page 118

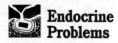

Pancreatic Disorders

Diabetes mellitus—*continued*

Expect the doctor to order fluid replacement, insulin therapy, electrolyte replacement, and antiacidosis therapy (if indicated).

Fluid replacement plays an important role. Rapid rehydration maintains vascular tone and metabolic function. The patient may have a 3- to 5-liter fluid deficit, so expect to administer large fluid amounts initially and to continue administration as needed. The solution you give depends on the patient's condition—usually, either hypotonic or normal saline solution. Expect to give 1,000 to 2,000 ml over the first 2 hours. When the glucose level slightly exceeds normal, the doctor may switch to a glucose solution, which helps prevent hypoglycemia and reduces the cerebral edema risk.

Insulin therapy begins once fluid replacement has been initiated. The patient with DKA needs immediate rapid-acting insulin to stop the pathologic cycle. The doctor will probably order small regular insulin doses, given I.V., I.M., or via a combination of methods, depending on the patient's condition. Usually, he'll order an initial I.V. bolus followed by continuous infusion. Monitor the patient's blood glucose level continuously during insulin infusion. When it reaches about 250 to 300 mg/dl, the doctor will probably decrease the insulin dose to prevent hypoglycemia. Typically, insulin decreases blood glucose levels by about 75 to 100 mg/dl each hour. Once the patient emerges from the initial hyperglycemic crisis, expect the doctor to resume the patient's usual insulin regimen.

Electrolyte replacement helps restore sodium, potassium, chloride, magnesium, and phosphate levels. Electrolyte supplements may be added to I.V. solutions. The hypotonic or normal saline solution you administer initially replaces sodium and chloride, but potassium replacement can be more difficult. Monitor serum electrolyte values as ordered, but keep in mind that the patient's serum potassium level doesn't reflect his true potassium balance, since most potassium remains within cells. DKA reduces the body's *total* potassium amount, although the patient's *serum* potassium level may be high, low, or even normal. If the potassium level's high, stay alert for hyperkalemia with life-threatening complications. When you administer insulin and fluids, potassium moves back into cells rapidly. The result may be life-threatening hypokalemia. The doctor will evaluate the need for potassium replacement carefully, using serum potassium levels as a guide. A high initial level indicates no need for potassium. A normal initial level suggests a need for potassium replacement (20 to 40 mEq/liter) after initial fluid replacement. As ordered, obtain an EKG to further evaluate the patient's potassium status. Peaked T waves, widened QRS complexes, and, sometimes, absent P waves indicate hyperkalemia. Prolonged QT intervals, depressed T waves, and prominent U waves indicate hypokalemia.

Antiacidosis therapy with bicarbonate may be necessary for a patient with an extremely low pH level. For most patients, however, fluid and insulin replacement alone usually correct metabolic acidosis.

Hyperglycemic hyperosmolar nonketotic coma (HHNC). Also known as hyperosmolar coma or hyperosmolar nonketotic coma, this emergency condition causes impaired consciousness—typically, coma or near-coma. The patient doesn't develop ketonemia for reasons that remain unclear. Clinical effects result from severe hyperglycemia

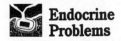
Pancreatic Disorders

(blood glucose levels above 800 mg/dl), hyperosmolarity (serum osmolarity of 280 mOsm/liter or higher), and severe dehydration from osmotic diuresis.

HHNC typically occurs in middle-aged or elderly patients, as diabetes' first appearance or as a severe exacerbation of previously mild, non-insulin-dependent diabetes. The patient usually develops polyuria and polydipsia, then suffers these other signs and symptoms:
- altered level of consciousness
- severe dehydration
- hypotension
- rapid respirations
- GI disturbances (abdominal discomfort, nausea, vomiting, ileus, and/or gastric stasis)
- signs of hypovolemic shock (in some cases).

Because it's usually not diagnosed early enough for effective treatment, HHNC has a high mortality. The doctor will make the diagnosis from the patient's clinical status and from laboratory tests revealing extremely elevated blood glucose levels without acetone.

Various acute and chronic illnesses or other conditions can precipitate HHNC by causing stress, which increases the patient's insulin needs. These conditions include:
- previously undiagnosed diabetes
- acute pancreatitis
- severe burns
- uremia
- dehydration
- thyrotoxicosis
- diabetes insipidus
- GI bleeding
- central nervous system damage
- acute pyelonephritis
- acute myocardial infarction
- gram-negative pneumonia
- subdural hematoma
- chronic renal insufficiency
- emotional distress.

In addition, the use of alcohol or certain drugs (including phenytoin [Dilantin], thiazide diuretics, steroids, mannitol, propranolol [Inderal], immunosuppressants, diazoxide, glucagon, furosemide [Lasix], ethacrynic acid [Edecrin], and cimetidine) may precipitate HHNC. Some medical procedures—peritoneal dialysis, I.V. hyperalimentation, prolonged mannitol-induced diuresis, nasogastric tube feedings with high-protein mixtures, and hypothermia—also increase the risk for HHNC.

Treatment for HHNC involves fluid replacement, insulin therapy, and electrolyte replacement.

Fluid replacement is even more important than insulin therapy for the patient with HHNC. Expect to give abundant I.V. fluids—hypotonic saline solution or, if the patient has hypovolemic shock, isotonic saline solution. (*Note:* If your patient's elderly, be sure to assess his fluid tolerance while you administer fluids.)

Continued on page 121

Pancreatic Disorders

Comparing hypoglycemia, DKA, and HHNC

Parameter	Hypoglycemia (insulin shock) Occurs in patients with or without diabetes mellitus	DKA Usually occurs in known Type I diabetic patients	HHNC Usually occurs in Type II diabetic patients (condition may be undiagnosed)
Precipitating factors	Delayed or omitted meal, insulin overdose, excessive exercise without food or insulin adjustments	Undiagnosed diabetes, neglected treatment, infection, cardiovascular disorders, physical stress, emotional distress	Undiagnosed diabetes, infection or other stress, acute or chronic illnesses, certain drugs and medical procedures, severe burns treated with high sugar concentrations
Symptom onset	Rapid (minutes to hours)	Slow (hours to days)	Slow (hours to days), but less gradual than DKA
Signs and symptoms			
Skin and mucous membranes	Cold, clammy skin; pallor; profuse sweating; normal mucous membranes	Warm, flushed, dry, loose skin; dry, crusty mucous membranes; soft eyeballs	Warm, flushed, dry, extremely loose skin; dry, crusty mucous membranes; soft eyeballs
Neurologic status	*Initial*—irritability, nervousness, giddiness; hand tremors; difficulty speaking, concentrating, focusing, and coordinating *Late*—hyperreflexia, dilated pupils, coma	*Initial*—dullness, confusion, lethargy; diminished reflexes *Late*—coma	*Initial*—dullness, confusion, lethargy, diminished reflexes *Late*—coma
Muscle strength	Normal or reduced	Extremely weak	Extremely weak
Gastrointestinal	None	Anorexia, nausea, vomiting, diarrhea, abdominal tenderness and pain	None
Temperature	Normal (subnormal if in deep coma)	Possible fever (from dehydration or infection)	Possible fever (from dehydration)
Pulse	Tachycardic (bradycardic in deep coma)	Mildly tachycardic, weak	Usually rapid
Blood pressure	Normal or above normal	Subnormal	Subnormal
Respirations	*Initial*—Normal to rapid *Late*—Slow	*Initial*—deep, fast *Late*—Kussmaul's	Rapid (but no Kussmaul's)
Breath odor	Normal	Fruity, acetone	Normal
Weight	Stable	Decreased	Decreased
Other	Hunger	Thirst	Thirst
Laboratory findings			
Blood glucose level	Below normal—below 70 mg/dl	Above normal	Markedly above normal
Serum sodium level	Normal	Normal or subnormal	Above normal, normal, or subnormal
Serum potassium level	Normal	Normal or above normal initially, then subnormal	Normal or above normal initially, then subnormal
Serum ketones	Negative	Positive/large	Negative/small
Serum osmolarity	Normal (290 to 310 mOsm/liter)	Above normal but usually less than 330 mOsm/liter	Markedly above normal—350 to 450 mOsm/liter
Hematocrit	Normal	Above normal	Above normal
Arterial blood gases	Normal or slight respiratory acidosis	Metabolic acidosis with compensatory respiratory alkalosis	Normal or slight metabolic acidosis
Urine glucose level	None	Above normal	Markedly above normal
Urine ketones	None	Positive/large	Negative/small
Urine output	Normal	*Initial*—polyuria *Late*—oliguria	Markedly above normal
Treatment	Glucose, glucagon, epinephrine	Insulin, fluid replacement, electrolyte replacement, antiacidosis therapy (if needed)	Fluid replacement, insulin, electrolyte replacement

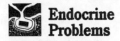
Pancreatic Disorders

Diabetes mellitus—*continued*

Insulin therapy immediately follows fluid replacement initiation. As ordered, give low insulin doses (usually by continuous I.V. infusion) to gradually decrease hyperglycemia and hyperosmolarity. Patients with HHNC have a greater insulin sensitivity than patients with DKA, so expect to give less insulin. Monitor blood glucose levels closely to help avoid hypoglycemia. When the blood glucose level approaches 250 mg/dl, expect to give I.V. glucose and to discontinue continuous I.V. insulin infusion. You may give further insulin subcutaneously, as ordered.

Electrolyte replacement aims to replace ions lost through osmotic diuresis. Normal saline solution replaces sodium and chloride; the doctor will consider parenteral potassium replacement after fluid replacement begins to shift potassium back to cells and lowers the serum potassium level. Then he may order potassium chloride or potassium phosphate added to the I.V. solution.

Other complications. Patients with diabetes mellitus have a higher risk for various chronic illnesses affecting virtually all body systems. The most common chronic complications include:
- cardiovascular disease
- peripheral vascular disease
- retinopathy
- nephropathy
- neuropathy.

Researchers don't know why these disorders particularly affect diabetics, but they do know that such complications usually appear about 10 years after diabetes mellitus' onset. They've also linked the incidence and severity of these complications with blood glucose control. Consequently, many doctors now advocate tight blood glucose control for diabetes management to prevent or minimize these complications.

Evaluation

Base your evaluation on the expected outcomes as listed on the nursing care plan. To determine if the patient's improved, ask yourself the following questions:
- Do the patient and his family understand the disease process?
- Can they identify signs and symptoms of hypoglycemia and hyperglycemia?
- Can the patient administer his insulin or sulfonylurea therapy properly? Does he know about the medication's potential adverse effects?
- Can he monitor his glucose level by urine or blood testing?
- Does he understand the need for good personal hygiene?
- Does he understand his dietary regimen?
- Do the patient and his family know about local diabetes mellitus support groups and how to contact them?

The answers to these questions will help you evaluate your patient's status and the effectiveness of his care. Keep in mind that these questions stem from the sample nursing care plan on page 104. Your questions may differ.

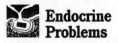
Pancreatic Disorders

Hypoglycemia

A symptom complex rather than a disease, hypoglycemia reflects abnormally low blood glucose levels leading to signs and symptoms that usually disappear when glucose returns to normal levels. Signs and symptoms depend on how rapidly blood glucose decreases, the initial blood glucose concentration, and the patient's sex (for unknown reasons, women usually have lower blood glucose levels than men). Blood glucose levels below 50 mg/dl usually produce signs and symptoms, although this varies greatly. A rapid blood glucose drop produces adrenergic signs and symptoms from excessive catecholamines released to counteract hypoglycemia. A gradual blood glucose fall produces neuroglycopenic signs and symptoms from gradual brain cell glucose deprivation.

Glucose derives mainly from food but can also be produced by hepatic glycogenolysis and gluconeogenesis. If blood glucose levels drop—either from sluggish glucose production or excessively rapid glucose removal (as by excessive insulin or exercise)—hypoglycemia occurs. Glucocorticoids, catecholamines, glucagon, and growth hormone normally stimulate endogenous glucose production through several different mechanisms; but a deficiency or disorder in any of these hormones can cause continued hypoglycemia (see *How hormones respond to hypoglycemia*).

Hypoglycemia types include reactive (also known as postprandial or fed), fasting, and pharmacologic.

Reactive hypoglycemia. This condition accounts for about 75% of spontaneous hypoglycemia cases. The patient typically has a normal fasting blood glucose level but develops symptomatic hypoglycemia within 5 hours after eating a meal. His signs and symptoms—predominantly adrenergic—usually appear mild and resolve quickly with treatment. Reactive hypoglycemia can take several different forms: reactive functional (idiopathic) hypoglycemia, alimentary

How hormones respond to hypoglycemia

Hormone	Secretion	Action	Effects
Epinephrine	Rapid	Rapid	• Increases hepatic glycogenolysis • Increases lipolysis • Decreases peripheral glucose utilization • Decreases insulin release
Glucagon	Rapid	Rapid	• Increases hepatic gluconeogenesis and glycogenolysis • Increases lipolysis
Glucocorticoids	Delayed	Probably immediate	• Increases hepatic gluconeogenesis • Increases lipolysis • Increases amino acid release from muscles • Decreases peripheral glucose utilization
Growth hormone	Delayed	Delayed	• Increases lipolysis • Decreases peripheral glucose utilization • Decreases insulin release

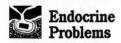
Pancreatic Disorders

hypoglycemia, and reactive hypoglycemia secondary to early Type II diabetes mellitus or impaired glucose tolerance.

In reactive functional hypoglycemia—the most common reactive hypoglycemia form—the patient has a rapid blood glucose drop 2 to 4 hours after a carbohydrate meal. Researchers haven't determined its mechanism but have linked this hypoglycemia type to a compulsive-perfectionistic personality with an intense achievement drive. Contrary to popular belief, reactive functional hypoglycemia doesn't predispose the patient to diabetes mellitus.

Alimentary hypoglycemia—also called late-stage dumping syndrome—reflects alimentary dysfunction, usually from extensive gastric surgery. Food enters the small bowel too rapidly, causing excessive glucose absorption. This produces hyperglycemia, which,

Continued on page 124

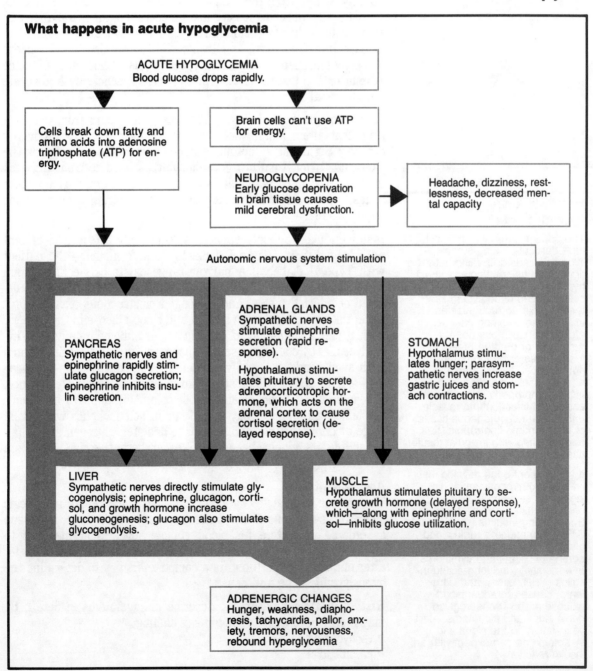

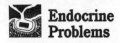
Pancreatic Disorders

Hypoglycemia—*continued*

in turn, stimulates excessive insulin release and subsequent hyperinsulinemia. Blood glucose levels fall abruptly 1 to 3 hours after eating.

In reactive hypoglycemia secondary to early Type II diabetes mellitus or impaired glucose tolerance, blood glucose levels fall abruptly 3 to 5 hours after a meal. The mechanism producing this rare condition may involve delayed insulin secretion.

Fasting hypoglycemia. In this condition, the patient's blood glucose level typically falls gradually, reaching an abnormally low level more than 5 hours after a meal. Neuroglycopenic signs and symptoms dominate, and the condition may be more severe and prolonged than reactive hypoglycemia. A rare disorder, fasting hypoglycemia usually results from liver disease or tumor formation. Insulinoma, for example, causes excessive insulin secretion; an extrapancreatic tumor leads to hypoglycemia through an unknown mechanism. Liver disease interferes with the liver's ability to raise blood glucose levels by gluconeogenesis and glycogenolysis. Other causes include adrenocortical insufficiency, growth hormone deficiency, and severe chronic renal failure.

Pharmacologic hypoglycemia. This disorder occurs from use of a drug that alters insulin secretion or the liver's glucose-producing capacity. Signs and symptoms depend on when the patient took the particular drug. Insulin and sulfonylureas used to treat diabetes mellitus (the most common causes), beta blockers, various other drugs, and excessive alcohol ingestion can all trigger pharmacologic hypoglycemia.

Insulin-induced hypoglycemia most commonly affects the patient with long-standing Type I diabetes; least commonly, the patient with Type II diabetes. A narrow range exists between optimum blood glucose levels and hypoglycemia; insulin dose changes, delayed or omitted meals, and prolonged or strenuous exercise may upset the balance between insulin and blood glucose in the diabetic patient (see *Insulin-induced hypoglycemia*). Sulfonylurea-induced hypoglycemia, by contrast, usually occurs in Type II diabetic patients with such conditions as liver disease, renal disease, or advanced age—all of which affect sulfonylurea metabolism and clearance. Alcohol-induced hypoglycemia most commonly appears in chronic alcoholics, although it may also occur in nonalcoholics who ingest large alcohol amounts and who have depleted glycogen stores (alcohol inhibits gluconeogenesis). Researchers theorize that beta blockers may cause hypoglycemia by inhibiting gluconeogenesis.

Assessment

The patient with acute hypoglycemia may have severe neurologic signs and symptoms that require emergency care. If so, intervene as ordered to restore his blood glucose level to normal and to alleviate signs and symptoms. If his clinical condition permits (or after initial treatment), obtain a complete history to determine the hypoglycemia type and cause.

History. Ask your patient to describe his symptoms in detail. He may report adrenergic symptoms, including:
- tachycardia
- palpitations

Insulin-induced hypoglycemia

The patient with diabetes mellitus—particulary long-standing Type I—treads a fine line between tight blood glucose control and hypoglycemia. Help him avoid insulin-induced hypoglycemia by teaching him to recognize and avoid these common causes:
- chronic insulin overdose
- delayed or omitted meals
- strenuous or prolonged exercise not balanced by extra calories
- faulty insulin injection techniques (improperly mixed insulin, accidental injection into muscle rather than subcutaneous tissue, or injection into lipotrophic sites or other sites with irregular insulin absorption).

If your patient does develop insulin-induced hypoglycemia, his signs and symptoms will depend on the insulin type he's taken. Short-acting insulins (regular and Semilente) cause a rapid blood glucose drop and corresponding adrenergic signs and symptoms. Intermediate- and long-acting insulins (NPH, Lente, and Ultralente) cause a gradual blood glucose drop with neuroglycopenic signs and symptoms. Alert your patient to the signs and symptoms he can expect with an insulin reaction.

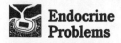
Pancreatic Disorders

Autoimmune hypoglycemia

First described in 1970, this rare hypoglycemia form arises secondarily to high levels of insulin-binding antibodies in patients who've never received exogenous insulin. Affected patients initially appear to have unusually high circulating insulin levels. However, this results from endogenous anti-insulin antibodies that compete with the insulin assay antibody, causing falsely high insulin levels. Researchers don't know the mechanism underlying autoimmune hypoglycemia, although they suspect the gradual, unregulated insulin release from a large circulating antibody-bound pool.

Hypoglycemia attacks may occur after eating or fasting; signs and symptoms may be adrenergic or neuroglycopenic. The syndrome's apparently unrelated to other autoimmune disorders, except with a few patients who've also had Graves' disease. Currently, doctors must rely on nonspecific therapy directed at hypoglycemia, although the syndrome sometimes resolves spontaneously.

* dizziness
* anxiety
* hunger
* nausea
* diaphoresis
* tremors
* pallor.

These symptoms—responses to the hormone release triggered by low blood glucose levels—usually appear with rapid blood glucose reduction. Typically, they represent early warning signs of impending cerebral impairment. As hypoglycemia continues, the brain's glucose supply suffers, resulting in neuroglycopenic signs and symptoms, such as:
* fatigue
* restlessness
* speech and motor dysfunction
* sleepiness
* headache
* visual changes, such as blurred vision
* mental status changes, such as confusion, bizarre behavior, and poor concentration
* focal neurologic signs.

If your patient reports any of these during your history taking, notify the doctor immediately. Prompt glucose restoration usually reverses these problems, but prolonged untreated hypoglycemia can cause coma, irreversible neurologic damage, and, ultimately, death.

Some patients who have long-standing diabetes mellitus with neuropathy and those who take drugs affecting the sympathetic nervous system (such as beta blockers) may not perceive early adrenergic symptoms. You may see such a patient only late in the hypoglycemic attack, when cerebral dysfunction alerts him or others. Or you may see him only after repeated hypoglycemic episodes.

The patient may have had recurrent hypoglycemic symptoms. Ask him how long the symptoms last each time—typically, they last from minutes to hours rather than from days to weeks. Blood glucose levels usually return to normal rapidly through counterregulatory mechanisms or food ingestion. If they don't, the patient will probably develop syncope, seizures, or coma as blood glucose levels continue to fall. Ask your patient if his symptoms disappear when he consumes glucose-containing foods or beverages, but remember that symptomatic relief with glucose ingestion doesn't confirm hypoglycemia.

To differentiate between reactive and fasting hypoglycemia, ask the patient when he last ate before his symptoms appeared:
* reactive functional hypoglycemia symptoms usually occur 2 to 4 hours after a meal
* alimentary hypoglycemia symptoms usually arise 1 to 3 hours after a meal
* symptoms of reactive hypoglycemia secondary to early Type II diabetes mellitus or impaired glucose tolerance usually occur 3 to 5 hours after a meal
* fasting hypoglycemia symptoms usually occur more than 5 hours after a meal.

Continued on page 126

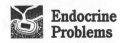
Pancreatic Disorders

Insulinomas: Functioning beta cell tumors

Pancreatic beta cells can give rise to benign or cancerous insulinomas (insulin-producing tumors). These rare tumors most commonly appear in patients aged 30 to 60. Because blood glucose levels decrease gradually, the patient usually has neuroglycopenic signs and symptoms of hypoglycemia—especially in the fasting state. He may have chronic lethargy and fatigue.

Small, autonomously functioning benign insulinomas—the most common insulinoma type—usually produce signs and symptoms related to excess insulin secretion rather than local tumor effects. Some insulinomas appear as multiple benign adenomas scattered throughout the pancreas.

Beta cell carcinomas—usually larger than adenomas and with a lower insulin content relative to weight—account for about 10% of beta cell tumors. These tumors may secrete hormones besides insulin, such as glucagon, gastrin, melanocyte-stimulating hormone, adrenocorticotropic hormone, vasopressin, secretin, and parathyroid hormone. Cancers that spread to regional lymph nodes and the liver typically cause death within about 3 years.

Assessment. Besides hypoglycemia signs and symptoms, the patient with a beta cell tumor has an inappropriately high insulin level. However, most tumors secrete excess insulin intermittently or only in slightly above-normal amounts. Therefore, the doctor must order multiple overnight fasting blood samples, prolonged fasting, or infusion of insulin secretagogues, such as tolbutamide or glucagon, to confirm the diagnosis. Proinsulin measurement also helps identify insulinomas. An above-normal proinsulin level suggests insulinoma.

Intervention. Expect the doctor to surgically remove the tumor after localizing it by subselective angiography. With an inoperable or recurrent cancerous insulinoma, hypoglycemia may persist. In this case, the doctor may order frequent high-carbohydrate feedings and oral diazoxide to maintain blood glucose levels. If these measures fail, he may order the anticancer drug streptozocin as palliative therapy.

Hypoglycemia—*continued*

Obtain a past medical history to help uncover more clues to hypoglycemia's cause. A history of gastric surgery (gastroenterostomy or partial or complete gastrectomy), impaired glucose tolerance, diabetes mellitus treated with insulin or sulfonylureas, excessive alcohol consumption, insulinoma, extrapancreatic tumor (especially a large mesothelioma, fibroma, fibrosarcoma, or leiomyosarcoma), or beta blocker use suggests the cause. Make sure you obtain a family and social history. The family history may reveal diabetes mellitus or hypoglycemia. The social history provides information about the patient's nutritional status and life-style.

Physical examination. Usually, the physical examination confirms adrenergic and, possibly, neuroglycopenic effects only in a patient who's currently suffering a hypoglycemic attack.

Diagnostic studies. In an emergency, you may check the patient's blood glucose levels with a monitoring strip such as a Chemstrip to help confirm suspected hypoglycemia. Remember, however, that this method may not reflect the patient's status accurately if it's performed incorrectly. Usually, the doctor will order laboratory analysis of the patient's blood glucose level. Draw a sample as ordered. The doctor will base his interventions on the patient's clinical condition rather than on the absolute blood glucose level, because each person responds differently to a given level.

The doctor may order an *oral glucose tolerance test* (usually a 5-hour study) if the patient's history suggests reactive hypoglycemia. This test detects abnormally low blood glucose levels in response to a glucose challenge, but it poses a risk for the patient with reactive functional hypoglycemia because he must eat a high-carbohydrate diet for 3 days before the test. The doctor may choose to defer the test and treat the patient's hypoglycemia based on his history alone.

If the patient's history suggests fasting hypoglycemia, the doctor may order concurrent fasting serum insulin and fasting glucose levels (taken during a 48- to 72-hour fast) to determine the serum insulin/glucose ratio. He may also order an I.V. glucose tolerance test. If the patient has an insulinoma or another tumor that secretes insulin or an insulin-like substance, these tests will reveal abnormally high insulin levels relative to glucose levels (see *Insulinomas: Functioning beta cell tumors*). A C-peptide assay helps distinguish fasting hypoglycemia caused by an insulinoma (elevated C-peptide level) from fasting hypoglycemia caused by exogenous insulin administration (normal C-peptide level).

Planning

Before determining your nursing care plan, develop the nursing diagnosis by identifying your patient's problem or potential problem, then relating it to its cause. Possible nursing diagnoses for a patient with hypoglycemia include:
- injury, potential for (altered cerebral function); related to inadequate blood glucose levels
- knowledge deficit; related to newly diagnosed disorder
- nutrition, alteration in (less than body requirements); related to hypoglycemia
- self-concept, disturbances in; related to chronic disease
- noncompliance; related to inadequate health care teaching
- fear; related to danger of hypoglycemic episode.

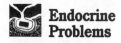
Pancreatic Disorders

Sample nursing care plan: Hypoglycemia

Nursing diagnosis	Expected outcomes
Injury, potential for (altered cerebral function); related to inadequate blood glucose levels	The patient will: • maintain an adequate blood glucose level. • lack signs and symptoms of altered cerebral function. • know how to recognize signs and symptoms of a hypoglycemic episode.

Nursing interventions	Discharge planning
• Observe patient for signs or symptoms of a hypoglycemic episode, such as altered cerebral function. • If a hypoglycemic episode occurs, protect patient from injury and be prepared to obtain a blood glucose sample and provide emergency treatment, such as by administering a fast-acting oral carbohydrate (orange juice or sugar), I.V. glucose (dextrose 50% solution), glucagon, or epinephrine, as ordered. • Provide appropriate diet and ensure adequate intake to prevent a hypoglycemic episode. • Discuss disease process and its signs and symptoms, treatment, and prevention with patient and his family. • If indicated, evaluate patient's skill in administering insulin and correct any errors.	• Reinforce patient and family instructions. • Teach patient and his family how to recognize hypoglycemia signs and symptoms. • Teach patient and his family how to administer emergency treatment if hypoglycemia occurs. Advise patient to carry fast-acting carbohydrate with him at all times. • Inform patient about preventive measures, if indicated. • Reinforce the need for complying with treatment and follow-up care. • Advise patient to avoid hazardous activities. • Teach patient and his family how to monitor blood glucose at home. • Advise patient to carry medical identification, such as a Medic Alert tag, at all times. • Advise patient when to seek medical care.

The sample care plan above shows expected outcomes, nursing interventions, and discharge planning for one nursing diagnosis listed on the opposite page. However, you'll want to tailor each care plan to the patient's needs.

Intervention

Treatment for hypoglycemia aims to restore and maintain normal blood glucose levels. Interventions include:
• emergency measures to increase blood glucose levels during an acute hypoglycemic episode
• long-term measures to help prevent hypoglycemia's recurrence.

Emergency measures. Treatment depends on the patient's symptoms—and may be needed even before you complete your assessment. If the patient's responsive, expect to give 10 to 15 g of a fast-acting oral carbohydrate initially or as ordered (see *Emergency hypoglycemia intervention*). If the patient's signs and symptoms persist after 15 minutes, expect to give an additional 10 g carbohydrate.

If the patient's unresponsive, give an I.V. bolus of dextrose 50% solution, as ordered, which should cause an immediate blood glucose increase. You may also give glucagon parenterally or epinephrine subcutaneously; both drugs raise blood glucose levels in a few minutes by stimulating glycogenolysis (provided liver glycogen stores haven't been depleted). *Don't* give glucagon to a patient whose hypoglycemia stems from chronic alcohol intoxication—his glycogen stores may be depleted. Instead, give I.V. thiamine, as ordered (to prevent an episode of Wernicke-Korsakoff syndrome); then expect to give dextrose. If possible, obtain a blood glucose sample before administering any glucose form.

Emergency hypoglycemia intervention

If your patient suffers an acute hypoglycemic attack, take these steps to help restore normal blood glucose levels and prevent complications:

If the patient's responsive—
Give a food or beverage containing 10 to 15 g of a simple, fast-acting carbohydrate. Possibilities include:
• ½ cup (4 oz) fruit juice, such as orange or apple juice
• ½ cup (4 oz) nondiet soft drink, such as ginger ale or cola
• ½ cup (4 oz) gelatin dessert
• 4 sugar cubes
• 2 sugar packets
• 2 graham cracker squares
• ¼ cup (2 oz) corn syrup, honey, or grape jelly
• 6 jelly beans
• 10 gumdrops.

If the patient's unresponsive—
Give medications as ordered. If these aren't available, squeeze a glucose product such as Glutose, Glutol, or Instant Glucose into the patient's mouth, where it can be absorbed through oral tissues or swallowed by reflex (but make sure you don't obstruct the patient's airway). If you can't obtain these products, place some honey on the patient's tongue, or squeeze prepared cake-decorating icing (such as CakeMate) between the patient's gum and cheeks. Obtain medical help promptly.

Continued on page 128

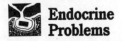
Pancreatic Disorders

Hypoglycemia—*continued*

Once the patient responds, assess him continuously and monitor his blood glucose levels, as ordered. Give him a complex-carbohydrate snack (such as peanut butter and crackers, cottage cheese and fruit, a small sandwich, or milk and graham crackers) when his signs and symptoms disappear to restore liver glycogen stores and to prevent hypoglycemia from recurring before the next mealtime.

Teach the patient and his family how to recognize and treat a hypoglycemic episode at home. Give the patient a list of fast-acting carbohydrates he should take if he develops symptoms, and advise him to carry hard candy or gumdrops. Tell him to keep glucagon at home, and make sure his family members know how and when to give it subcutaneously. Advise the patient to carry a medical identification card or tag (such as a Medic Alert bracelet) to ensure prompt treatment in case he becomes unresponsive. Tell him to contact his doctor if episodes become frequent or severe and to try to recall his activities before an acute attack to help identify the cause.

Long-term measures. Once the doctor determines hypoglycemia's underlying cause, he may treat it with diet, medication, or surgery, as indicated.

Diet therapy helps the patient who has fasting or reactive hypoglycemia. For fasting hypoglycemia, the doctor will order a diet that increases caloric intake so that the body's glucose supply balances the excessive insulin secretion. Tell the patient *never* to skip a meal—if he does, he may develop severe or prolonged hypoglycemia. For reactive hypoglycemia, the doctor will order frequent, small meals spread evenly throughout the day to prevent excessive insulin secretion. Usually, the diet includes abundant complex carbohydrates (such as pasta and bread), fiber, and fat and prohibits simple sugars, alcohol, fruit drinks, and caffeine. If the patient's obese and has reactive hypoglycemia secondary to early Type II diabetes mellitus, the doctor will probably prescribe a weight-reduction diet.

Medications used to treat hypoglycemia's underlying cause include:
• tranquilizers, such as diazepam, for the patient with reactive functional hypoglycemia (to help relieve tension and anxiety)
• anticholinergics for the patient with alimentary or reactive functional hypoglycemia (to delay gastric emptying and prevent excessive insulin secretion resulting from rapid glucose absorption)
• propranolol for the patient with reactive hypoglycemia (to alleviate adrenergic signs and symptoms)
• oral diazoxide for the patient with fasting hypoglycemia caused by an inoperable insulinoma (to inhibit insulin release)
• chemotherapy for the patient with fasting hypoglycemia from an inoperable insulinoma.

Teach your patient about his prescribed medication. Also advise him to avoid all over-the-counter medications unless approved by his doctor; many such drugs contain ingredients that lower blood glucose levels.

Surgery may be performed to remove an operable insulinoma or an extrapancreatic tumor causing excessive secretion of insulin or an insulin-like substance.

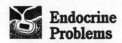
Pancreatic Disorders

Nursing interventions. Patient education and compliance can help control hypoglycemia regardless of the cause and type. Advise the patient with reactive or pharmacologic hypoglycemia to review his life-style to identify such precipitating factors as poor diet, stress, or poor compliance with his diabetes regimen. Explore ways to help the patient change or avoid these factors. If necessary, review stress-management techniques or encourage him to join a diabetes support group. For the patient with insulin-induced hypoglycemia, review diabetes management as necessary. Arrange for him to see his doctor regularly and to report all hypoglycemic episodes.

Evaluation

Base your evaluation on the expected outcomes as listed on the nursing care plan. To determine if the patient's improved, ask yourself the following questions:
• Does the patient have an adequate blood glucose level?
• Does he show signs and symptoms of inadequate cerebral function?
• Does he know how to prevent a hypoglycemic episode?
• Do the patient and his family know how to treat hypoglycemia if it occurs?

The answers to these questions will help you evaluate your patient's status and the effectiveness of his care. Keep in mind that these questions stem from the sample nursing care plan on page 127. Your questions may differ.

Self-Test

1. Counterregulatory hormones that help increase blood glucose levels include all of the following except:
a. cortisol   **b.** growth hormone   **c.** vasopressin   **d.** epinephrine

2. Which term refers to glucose formation from noncarbohydrates?
a. glycogenesis   **b.** glycogenolysis   **c.** glycolysis
d. gluconeogenesis

3. Classic diabetes mellitus signs and symptoms include all of the following except:
a. polyuria   **b.** polydipsia   **c.** polyphagia   **d.** polyopia

4. Which of the following insulin types has a short duration of action?
a. Semilente Insulin   **b.** NPH Insulin   **c.** Humulin N   **d.** PZI Iletin I

5. If your patient has fasting hypoglycemia, he may have all of the following signs and symptoms except:
a. below-normal blood glucose level within 5 hours after a meal
b. behavioral changes   **c.** motor incoordination   **d.** headache

Answers (page number shows where answer appears in text)
1. **c** (page 91)   2. **d** (page 91)   3. **d** (page 93)   4. **a** (page 106)
5. **a** (page 124)

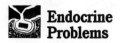
Adrenal Disorders: Cushing's Syndrome, Adrenocortical Insufficiency, and Other Problems

Christine A. Kessler wrote this chapter. Ms. Kessler is Assistant Professor, School of Health Sciences, Seattle Pacific University. She received her BSN and MSN from the University of Washington, Seattle. She is also a certified CCRN.

Adrenal gland dysfunction causes adrenal hormone excess or deficit. Because adrenal hormones produce widespread effects, such dysfunction may create a confusing clinical picture. Signs and symptoms—possibly acute or chronic—may mimic disorders of vastly different origins. Thus, diagnosis may prove difficult. Yet survival may depend on prompt detection and intervention. By enhancing your knowledge of adrenal pathophysiology, you can provide better care for a patient with an adrenal disorder.

Before studying these disorders, take the time to read *Reviewing adrenal gland structure and function.* Then review the additional information on adrenal function on the next few pages.

The adrenal glands produce the following hormones: glucocorticoids (most importantly, cortisol); mineralocorticoids (most importantly, aldosterone); catecholamines (epinephrine and norepinephrine); and androgens and estrogens (in small amounts). Glucocorticoids and mineralocorticoids collectively go by the name corticosteroids.

The adrenal glands contain two distinct regions—cortex and medulla. Each region has separate functions.

Adrenocortical function. The adrenal cortex secretes the body's total glucocorticoid and mineralocorticoid supply as well as some androgens and estrogens.

Glucocorticoid, androgen, and estrogen secretion depend on adrenocortical stimulation by adrenocorticotropic hormone (ACTH), produced by the anterior pituitary gland. Corticotropin-releasing factor, produced by the brain's hypothalamus, controls ACTH release into the bloodstream. Three factors regulate ACTH secretion: circulating cortisol levels, stress, and circadian rhythms (diurnal variation). Related to sleep-wake cycles, circadian rhythms may vary with daily activity changes. ACTH release usually peaks between 6 a.m. and 7 a.m. Cortisol secretion follows, peaking at about 8 a.m., dropping at about noon, and falling lowest between 9 p.m. and midnight.

Normal adrenocortical functioning requires an intact hypothalamic-pituitary axis. Circulating cortisol levels respond directly to a feedback system involving ACTH: As serum cortisol levels decline, ACTH release increases, and vice versa. Stressful physical, emotional, and environmental stimuli also trigger ACTH release and a subsequent serum cortisol increase. Although this so-called stress response remains poorly understood, it produces obvious benefits. For example, glucocorticoids released during stress promote metabolism of such vital substances as protein, amino acids, fatty acids, and glucose.

A much different process controls mineralocorticoids. Renin-angiotensin system activation, regulated by the kidney's juxtaglomerular apparatus, primarily governs aldosterone release. Initial renin secretion usually occurs in response to blood volume, blood pressure, and serum sodium level reductions. Through a complex process, renin release leads to angiotensin II production, which then stimulates aldosterone formation. The higher the angiotensin level, the

Continued on page 133

Adrenal Disorders

Reviewing adrenal gland structure and function

The adrenal glands—flat, pyramid-shaped structures—lie atop each kidney, surrounded by a thick fibrous capsule that supports their delicate tissues. Each gland weighs between 3 and 6 g and measures 1⅝″ to 2⅜″ (4 to 6 cm) long. (*Note:* The adrenal glands are also called the suprarenal glands.)

The adrenal glands have two portions—cortex and medulla—which share few features other than their adjacent housing within the retroperitoneal cavity. These structures originate from different embryonic tissue—the cortex from the mesoderm (from which reproductive glands develop); the medulla from the ectoderm (from which the sympathetic nervous system arises). Their functions relate closely to their respective origins.

The adrenal cortex, firm and golden yellow, completely encloses the medulla and accounts for about four fifths of the gland's bulk. Each of its three histologic zones secretes specific hormones. The outermost layer, the *glomerular zone,* secretes mineralocorticoids, with aldosterone the most potent. Mineralocorticoids help regulate fluid and electrolyte balance. The middle layer, or *fascicular zone,* produces glucocorticoids—most notably, cortisol, which plays a key role in the body's

immune response as well as in glucose and protein metabolism. The innermost layer, the *reticular zone,* produces some glucocorticoids and, along with the fascicular zone, may also produce androgens (such as testosterone) and small estrogen amounts.

The soft, reddish brown adrenal medulla contains irregularly arranged chromaffin cells that produce, secrete, and store catecholamines. Together, the medulla and the sympathetic nervous system form an anatomic and physiologic unit called the sympathoadrenal system. The splanchnic nerve supplies the medulla's sympathetic stimulation.

Adrenal blood supply comes from the renal arteries or directly from the abdominal aorta. After entering the gland, blood vessels become sinusoids, supplying both the cortex and medulla. The right adrenal gland drains directly into the vena cava; the left adrenal gland, into the left renal vein.

In conjunction with the nervous system and other endocrine glands, the adrenal glands contribute to homeostasis, allowing physical and emotional adaptation to internal and external changes. Thus, they're crucial to metabolism, the body's stress response, and fluid and electrolyte balance.

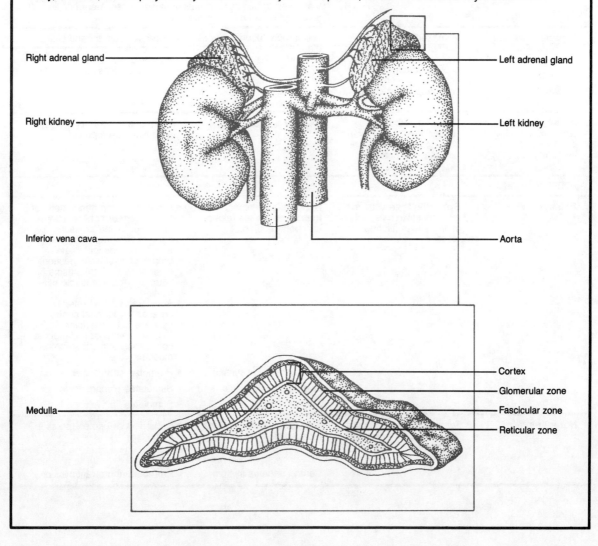

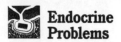
Adrenal Disorders

Adrenal hormones

Hormone	Releasing/inhibiting stimulus	Primary target site	Primary effects
ADRENAL CORTEX			
Glucocorticoids (such as cortisol)	Adrenocorticotropic hormone (ACTH) levels	Hypothalamic-pituitary axis	• Helps regulate ACTH secretion through negative feedback mechanism
		Kidney tubules	• Helps maintain fluid and electrolyte balance by promoting sodium and water retention and potassium excretion
		All body cells	• Promotes protein catabolism by stimulating protein breakdown and inhibiting protein synthesis
		Peripheral tissue	• Modifies glucose metabolism by increasing glucogenolysis and decreasing glucose uptake
		Adipose tissue	• Enhances fat deposition, especially in the abdomen, back, face, and supraclavicular areas
		Note: A glucocorticoid *excess* acts on all body tissues by suppressing inflammatory and immune responses as it stabilizes lysosomal membranes, reduces prostaglandin production and capillary permeability, and interferes with leukocyte migration to areas of inflammation, phagocytosis, and cell-mediated immunity. An excess also affects the hematologic system by stimulating erythropoiesis or causing leukocytosis, neutrophilia, lymphocytopenia, or eosinopenia.	
Mineralocorticoids (such as aldosterone)	Increased serum potassium concentration, decreased plasma volume, decreased sodium concentration, and/or renin-angiotensin system activation	Distal renal tubules, sweat glands, salivary glands, and intestines	• Increases sodium and water reabsorption (by expanding extracellular volume) • Increases potassium excretion
Androgens (such as testosterone; also small estrogen amounts)	ACTH and other factors; secreted intermittently in conjunction with cortisol, with marked increase during puberty	All body tissues	• Promotes secondary sex characteristic development
ADRENAL MEDULLA			
Epinephrine	Sympathetic nervous system stimulation, especially during stress (flight or fight reaction)	Heart muscle, smooth muscle, arterioles (alpha- and beta-receptors)	• Produces sympathomimetic effects (flight or fight reaction)—increases blood pressure, oxygen consumption, and carbon dioxide production; dilates bronchioles; slows digestion; postpones skeletal muscle fatigue (increases muscle efficiency) • Accelerates heart rate, increases myocardial contractility, constricts arterioles (pressor response), stimulates contraction of most smooth muscles
		Central nervous system	• Promotes neurotransmission
		Liver, skeletal muscle	• Stimulates glycogenesis
		Adipose tissue	• Stimulates lipolysis
Norepinephrine	Sympathetic nervous system stimulation, especially during stress (flight or fight reaction)	Arterioles (primarily alpha receptors)	• Constricts arterioles (pressor response)
		Central nervous system	• Promotes neurotransmission

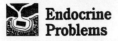
Adrenal Disorders

Continued

more aldosterone produced. Precisely how angiotensin II promotes aldosterone synthesis remains unknown.

Serum potassium and sodium levels also directly affect aldosterone release. Elevated serum potassium levels increase aldosterone secretion, and vice versa. Serum sodium levels have the opposite effect, with low levels increasing aldosterone release, and vice versa. ACTH has little regulatory effect on aldosterone (see *Corticosteroid secretion* for details).

Adrenomedullary function. Chromaffin cells in the adrenal medulla produce and secrete the catecholamines epinephrine (adrenaline) and norepinephrine (noradrenaline), as well as minute dopamine

Continued on page 134

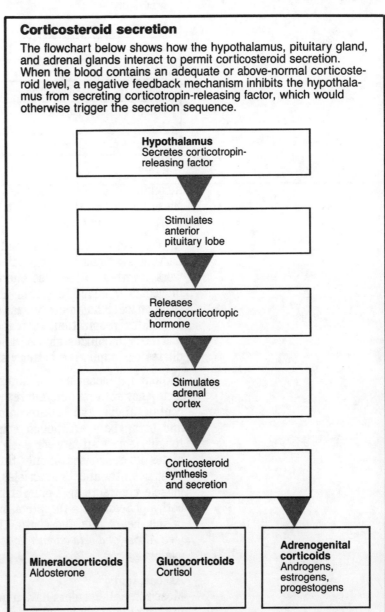

Corticosteroid secretion

The flowchart below shows how the hypothalamus, pituitary gland, and adrenal glands interact to permit corticosteroid secretion. When the blood contains an adequate or above-normal corticosteroid level, a negative feedback mechanism inhibits the hypothalamus from secreting corticotropin-releasing factor, which would otherwise trigger the secretion sequence.

Hypothalamus
Secretes corticotropin-releasing factor

↓

Stimulates anterior pituitary lobe

↓

Releases adrenocorticotropic hormone

↓

Stimulates adrenal cortex

↓

Corticosteroid synthesis and secretion

↓

Mineralocorticoids
Aldosterone

Glucocorticoids
Cortisol

Adrenogenital corticoids
Androgens, estrogens, progestogens

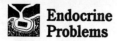
Adrenal Disorders

Alpha- and beta-adrenergic stimulation: Comparing catecholamine-induced effects

Parameter	Alpha stimulation	Beta₁ stimulation	Beta₂ stimulation
Vascular bed	Vasoconstriction (except in cardiac and skeletal muscles)	No effect	Vasodilation
Bronchial smooth muscle	No effect	No effect	Relaxation
Intestinal smooth muscle	No effect	No effect	Relaxation
Cardiac contractility	No effect	Increase	No effect
Heart rate	No effect	Increase	No effect
Pupils	Dilation	No effect	No effect
Perspiration	Increase	No effect	No effect
Skin	Piloerection	No effect	No effect
Insulin	Inhibits release	No effect	Stimulates release
Blood glucose	Increase	No effect	Decrease

Continued

amounts. Because the sympathetic nervous system also secretes these hormones, the adrenal medulla can be removed without impairing body function.

In response to acute stress and perceived danger, the sympathetic nervous system stimulates catecholamine release. Catecholamines work together to increase energy to cells, thus helping the body immediately adapt to stress. For example, in the flight or fight reaction, catecholamine release stimulates cardiovascular function, facilitates respiration, increases muscular capacity, intensifies alertness, mobilizes glucose and fatty acids, reduces fatigue, and dilates the pupils (for better vision).

Although epinephrine and norepinephrine each produce similar effects, they activate different receptors. Target-organ cell membranes contain alpha- and beta-receptors, subdivided into alpha₁, alpha₂, and beta₁, beta₂. Although epinephrine and norepinephrine have roughly equal affinity for each receptor type, norepinephrine mediates its responses mainly through alpha-receptors. This action most potently affects arterioles, causing vasoconstriction (smooth muscle contraction). Epinephrine mediates its responses through both alpha- and beta-receptors, but more potently mediates the latter, raising heart rate and contractility and relaxing smooth muscles (see *Alpha- and beta-adrenergic stimulation: Comparing catecholamine-induced effects*).

Assessment

Most adrenal disorders have a gradual onset and slow progression. In early stages, clinical changes may be too subtle to detect. Because glucocorticoids modify energy metabolism and muscle function,

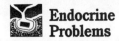
Adrenal Disorders

abnormal serum glucocorticoid levels may lead to such problems as weight changes, fatigue, and apathy—vague symptoms that may suggest various other causes. Some patients may be labeled as depressed, malingering, or neurotic, leaving the underlying adrenal problem undiagnosed. By the time later signs and symptoms, such as appearance changes, become obvious, treatment may prove ineffective.

To detect adrenal dysfunction early, stay alert for both subjective and objective clues as you take the patient's history and perform the physical examination. Note any reported or observed changes in mental acuity, emotional stability, activity tolerance, weight, appetite, skin, and libido. (For more information on assessing for a specific adrenal disorder, see the information under that disorder.)

History. Begin your assessment by obtaining a thorough health history. The patient with adrenal dysfunction will probably have a nonspecific chief complaint, such as fatigue, weakness, weight change, pigmentation changes, or nervousness. To investigate your patient's present illness, ask such questions as the following:

Have your problems affected your life-style? If so, have you taken any measures to relieve them? Have you experienced increasing fatigue, weakness, or lethargy? How much activity can you tolerate? At what time of day do you feel most fatigued? Has your sleep pattern changed? Have you had a gradual or sudden weight gain or loss? Have you had more infections or colds than usual? Have you had many headaches recently? How often and what type? Have you noticed any visual changes, such as blurred or double vision?

Have you had any difficulty breathing, especially during exertion or when lying down? (This may indicate increased fluid volume from adrenocortical hyperfunction.) Have you had palpitations? (This suggests pheochromocytoma.) Do you get dizzy or faint on rising from a reclining position? (Adrenocortical deficiency may produce fluid volume depletion leading to orthostatic hypotension.)

Have you felt depressed, irritable, unusually euphoric, or apathetic? Do you feel anxious, nervous, or confused? Have you noticed any tremors, especially with increased fatigue? Have you had numbness or tingling in your face or extremities? (This suggests aldosteronism, which may precipitate hypocalcemia.)

Have you had any bone pain, joint aches, or muscle cramps? Does the problem seem generalized or localized? What seems to exacerbate it? What seems to relieve it?

Has your overall appearance changed? Have you noticed any skin changes, such as increased or decreased pigmentation, increased perspiration, easy bruising, swelling (especially around the ankles), excessive hair loss, or body hair increase or abnormal distribution? Do your wounds seem to take longer to heal or become easily infected?

Obtain information about the patient's past medical and surgical history. Also ask about childhood growth and developmental patterns. Record any medication he's taking (prescribed or over-the-counter); especially note those containing steroids. For a woman,

Continued on page 136

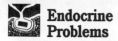
Adrenal Disorders

Continued

ask about her obstetric history and find out at what age she began menstruating. Also note when her last menstrual period began.

Ask the patient if he has a family history of endocrine disorders, growth or weight abnormalities, or hirsutism (to help distinguish true adrenal abnormality from familial tendency).

Adrenal disorders worsen with stress, so be sure to ask your patient about any recent stressful conditions at work or home. Also try to identify your patient's usual coping patterns.

Determine your patient's nutritional status by asking him the following questions: Has your appetite decreased lately? How much food do you eat on an average day? What types of foods do you eat? What's your average daily or weekly alcohol intake? Have you had any recent nausea, vomiting, diarrhea, constipation, or heartburn? Do you crave or use much salt? Has your thirst increased lately? How much fluid do you drink each day?

To identify the patient's elimination habits, ask if he's been urinating more frequently lately. Find out how often he urinates and whether he wakes up during the night to urinate.

Also ask about any recent libido changes or sexual dysfunction. With a woman, find out if she's had any menstrual cycle changes.

As you take your patient's history, also evaluate his mental acuity, behavior, and speech patterns to help determine his teaching needs.

Physical examination. Although you can't examine the adrenal glands themselves by inspection, palpation, percussion, or auscultation, you can assess the patient's physical appearance for clues to possible adrenal dysfunction. Does he appear alert and actively responsive to you and the surrounding environment? Observe his posture and facial expression. Do they convey vigor and vitality or fatigue, apathy, withdrawal, and discomfort? Does his weight seem appropriate for his height and body frame? Does he have abnormal or absent secondary sex characteristics? Do the external genitalia seem appropriate to sex? Signs of masculinization in a woman suggest excessive adrenal androgen production.

Observe for delayed or stunted growth, which may indicate congenital adrenal hyperplasia. Next, note body fat distribution. If your patient's obese, does his fat appear evenly distributed, with some concentration in the buttocks, lower abdomen, and inner thighs? This suggests ordinary obesity. Fat concentrated in the face and neck, interscapular region, trunk, and pelvic girdle suggests Cushing's syndrome—especially if the patient has thin arms and legs.

Next, examine your patient's skin. Poor skin turgor may mean dehydration from adrenocortical insufficiency. Look for multiple bruised areas, unhealed lesions, or purplish striae on the abdomen, breasts, and upper thighs. These findings commonly accompany Cushing's syndrome, which causes excess protein catabolism and impaired collagen formation. Assess for pitting edema, especially in dependent areas such as the ankles and sacral region. This may

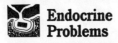
Adrenal Disorders

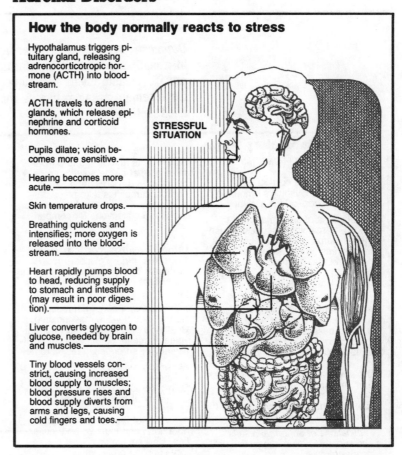

How the body normally reacts to stress

Hypothalamus triggers pituitary gland, releasing adrenocorticotropic hormone (ACTH) into bloodstream.

ACTH travels to adrenal glands, which release epinephrine and corticoid hormones.

Pupils dilate; vision becomes more sensitive.

Hearing becomes more acute.

Skin temperature drops.

Breathing quickens and intensifies; more oxygen is released into the bloodstream.

Heart rapidly pumps blood to head, reducing supply to stomach and intestines (may result in poor digestion).

Liver converts glycogen to glucose, needed by brain and muscles.

Tiny blood vessels constrict, causing increased blood supply to muscles; blood pressure rises and blood supply diverts from arms and legs, causing cold fingers and toes.

STRESSFUL SITUATION

result from aldosteronism or Cushing's syndrome, which leads to abnormal water and sodium retention.

Skin pigmentation can also help determine adrenal function. Check for generalized or localized hyperpigmentation—a hallmark of Addison's disease. Because hyperpigmentation can range from tan to brown, be sure to consider possible ethnic variations. Localized pigmentation usually appears in palm creases, gums, nipples, and scars. Occasionally, patchy hypopigmentation areas (vitiligo) may occur.

Check for hair distribution changes. Adrenocortical hyperfunction can cause excessive body hair (hirsutism) and make head hair sparse and easily pluckable.

Nearly all adrenal disorders cause muscle weakness. Assess muscle strength and tone by having your patient flex and extend his legs, arms, or head as you apply moderate counterresistance. Note the degree and symmetry of any muscle atrophy. Observe for tremors and paresthesia.

Make sure you assess the patient's vital signs. Does he have chronic or paroxysmal hypertension? Does his blood pressure drop when he moves from a reclining to an upright or standing position? Do you detect accompanying tachycardia or bradycardia?

Because other endocrine abnormalities may accompany an adrenal disorder, also evaluate your patient's thyroid, pancreas, and pituitary function.

Continued on page 138

Adrenal Disorders

Continued

Diagnostic studies. Like other hormones, adrenal hormones appear in minute amounts in body fluids, requiring highly sensitive and precise measurement techniques. Radioimmunoassay, also called displacement assay, ranks as the most precise and most commonly used method.

Selected laboratory tests

ADRENAL CORTEX FUNCTION TESTS
Serum cortisol
Measures serum cortisol levels; helps assess Cushing's syndrome and adrenocortical insufficiency

Implications of abnormal results:
Above-normal value suggests Cushing's syndrome but may also result from stress (such as from acute illness, trauma, or surgery). Normal or below-normal value occurs with adrenocortical insufficiency.

Nursing considerations:
• As ordered, draw blood samples at 8 a.m. and again at 4 p.m. or 8 p.m. (to assess circadian rhythm—related changes); 8 a.m. value usually equals twice the 8 p.m. value.

Dexamethasone suppression test
Screening test; helps diagnose Cushing's syndrome and differentiates adrenocortical hyperplasia from adrenal tumor

Implications of abnormal results:
Above-normal value suggests Cushing's syndrome.

Nursing considerations:
• Test may be performed as low-dose overnight test (most common), low-dose 2-day test, or high-dose test. In low-dose overnight test, patient receives 1 mg dexamethasone orally at midnight. Blood sampling takes place at 8 a.m. the next day.
• Doctor may order bedtime sedative to ensure a good night's rest.
• False-positive result may occur in patient who's extremely ill or anxious or who's taking an interfering drug, such as phenytoin (Dilantin) or estrogen.

Adrenocorticotropic hormone (ACTH) stimulation test
Helps screen for adrenocortical insufficiency

Implications of abnormal results:
Normally, serum cortisol level doubles and urinary 17-hydroxycorticosteroid (17-OHCS) level rises four to five times above baseline. Little or no response suggests primary adrenocortical insufficiency. Levels may remain normal with secondary adrenocortical insufficiency or chronic iatrogenic adrenal suppression.

Nursing considerations:
• Test may be performed by either method described below:
—Baseline serum cortisol sampling takes place 20 minutes before patient receives 250 mcg ACTH I.M., then again 30 minutes and 60 minutes after ACTH administration.
—Patient receives I.V. infusion of

ACTH or its analog (25 to 50 U/500 ml in normal saline solution) over 8 hours for 3 days. Routine serum cortisol samplings take place concomitantly with three 24-hour urine 17-OHCS collections for comparison.

Urine 17-hydroxycorticosteroids
Measures urinary glucocorticoids; evaluates cortisol secretion and indirectly assesses adrenocortical function

Implications of abnormal results:
Above-normal value may indicate Cushing's syndrome. Below-normal value suggests adrenocortical insufficiency or adrenogenital syndrome.

Nursing considerations:
• Adrenal glands normally secrete 20 mg cortisol daily; the body excretes about half as urinary 17-OHCS.
• Throw out first-voided specimen, note time, and start 24-hour collection. Chill specimen or use laboratory-supplied preservative.

Urine 17-ketosteroids (17-KS)
Evaluates adrenocortical function

Implications of abnormal results:
Above-normal level suggests primary or secondary Cushing's syndrome or adrenogenital syndrome. Below-normal level may occur with myxedema, exogenous steroid use, or starvation.

Nursing considerations:
• Obtain 24-hour collection (typically in conjunction with adrenal stimulation and suppression tests).

Metyrapone test
Evaluates pituitary-adrenal feedback mechanism; distinguishes adrenocortical hyperplasia from adrenal tumor

Implications of abnormal results:
17-OHCS value two to four times above normal indicates secondary Cushing's syndrome.

Nursing considerations:
• Patient receives 750 mg metyrapone (which blocks cortisol synthesis) every 4 hours for 24 hours. Obtain 24-hour urine collection for 17-OHCS before, during, and after metyrapone administration.
• ACTH stimulation test may be performed before metyrapone test begins to assess adrenal responsiveness to ACTH.
• Stay alert for signs and symptoms of adrenal insufficiency caused by metyrapone administration.

• Give metyrapone with food to prevent such adverse effects as nausea and vertigo.

ADRENAL MEDULLA FUNCTION TESTS
Serum catecholamines
Screens for pheochromocytoma

Implications of abnormal results:
Value three to four times above normal suggests pheochromocytoma.

Nursing considerations:
• Test has less diagnostic value than urinary catecholamine test.
• Have patient lie supine during test.
• Provide for restful, comfortable environment for 30 to 40 minutes before test, because anxiety can elevate test results.

Urinary vanillylmandelic acid (VMA)
Measures urinary catecholamine metabolites; screens for pheochromocytoma

Implications of abnormal results:
Above-normal value suggests pheochromocytoma.

Nursing considerations:
• Obtain 24-hour urine collection and keep it at pH of 3 or less by adding hydrochloric acid as preservative.
• Use of such drugs as methyldopa, reserpine, salicylates, and bronchodilators can elevate values. If possible, discontinue these drugs 3 days before testing.
• Advise patient to avoid coffee, tea, vanilla extract, chocolate, and bananas for 3 days before test—these foods can cause false elevations.

Urine metanephrines
Measures metanephrines (epinephrine metabolites); screens for pheochromocytoma

Implications of abnormal results:
Above-normal value suggests pheochromocytoma.

Nursing considerations:
• Test gives slightly more specific results than urinary VMA test.
• Obtain 24-hour urine collection and keep specimens at pH of 3 or less by adding hydrochloric acid as preservative.
• Use of such drugs as methyldopa, reserpine, salicylates, and bronchodilators can elevate values. If possible, discontinue these drugs 3 days before test.
• Advise patient to avoid coffee, tea, vanilla extract, chocolate, and bananas for 3 days before test—these foods can cause false elevations.

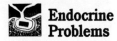

Adrenal Disorders

Laboratory evaluation of a patient with an adrenal problem starts with baseline adrenal hormone measurements. If these tests reveal abnormalities, the doctor will order more definitive studies to pinpoint the disorder. For example, if he suspects adrenal hypofunction, he'll probably order an ACTH stimulation test to determine whether the primary problem lies within the adrenal cortex or the anterior pituitary lobe. Serum cortisol that remains at baseline level in response to administered ACTH suggests primary adrenocortical hypofunction.

Remember—hormone measurement reflects the hormone level only at sampling time. Because adrenal hormone secretion fluctuates throughout the day, expect the doctor to order repeated measurements (such as 24-hour collections) rather than random samplings for more reliable results.

Anxiety and stress can alter adrenal hormone secretion and may reduce test accuracy. When preparing your patient for diagnostic testing, try to reduce his anxiety by encouraging him to express his concerns. Explain the test's purpose and procedure so he'll know what to expect, and assure him that the test doesn't cause pain.

If you're responsible for test scheduling, you can help improve test accuracy by considering how circadian rhythm affects some adrenal hormone levels. For example, because cortisol levels normally peak in the early morning and ebb in the evening, peak and baseline serum cortisol levels should be drawn at 8 a.m. and 8 p.m., respectively. (See *Selected laboratory tests* for more information on adrenal hormone tests.)

Cushing's syndrome

Cushing's syndrome (also called hypercortisolism) reflects a glucocorticoid excess—in particular, a cortisol excess. Depending on the disorder's cause, excessive mineralocorticoids and androgens may also be secreted. The disorder affects more women than men.

Cushing's syndrome can be primary, secondary, or iatrogenic. *Primary Cushing's syndrome* stems from an intrinsic adrenocortical disorder (commonly, a neoplasm). *Secondary Cushing's syndrome* (also called Cushing's disease) results from pituitary or hypothalamic dysfunction that causes increased ACTH secretion and subsequent glucocorticoid excess. Adrenal hyperplasia accompanies secondary Cushing's syndrome.

Iatrogenic Cushing's syndrome usually stems from excessive or chronic administration of synthetic steroids with glucocorticoid activity (such as cortisone or prednisone). Such drugs enjoy widespread use because of their anti-inflammatory and immunosuppressive effects. By artificially elevating cortisol levels, they suppress ACTH secretion, causing adrenal atrophy. Consequently, although the patient may have signs and symptoms of adrenal hyperfunction, acute adrenal insufficiency can occur suddenly with abrupt steroid withdrawal.

Assessment

When assessing a patient for Cushing's syndrome, keep in mind that the disorder causes exaggerated glucocorticoid effects, re-

Comparing Cushing's disease and Cushing's syndrome

Cushing's disease: Glucocorticoid excess resulting from pituitary adrenocorticotropic hormone hypersecretion

Cushing's syndrome: Glucocorticoid excess from any cause

Continued on page 140

Adrenal Disorders

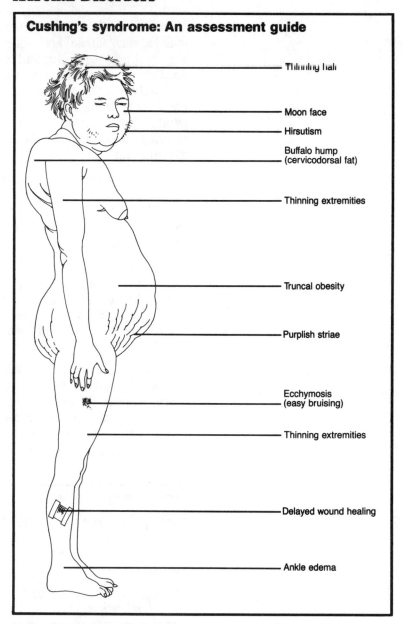

Cushing's syndrome: An assessment guide

- Thinning hair
- Moon face
- Hirsutism
- Buffalo hump (cervicodorsal fat)
- Thinning extremities
- Truncal obesity
- Purplish striae
- Ecchymosis (easy bruising)
- Thinning extremities
- Delayed wound healing
- Ankle edema

Cushing's syndrome—*continued*

flected by fluid and electrolyte disturbances, metabolic disorders, altered fat distribution, and suppressed immune response. A concomitant androgen excess may lead to hirsutism and virilization.

History. Begin your assessment by determining the patient's chief complaint. He may report fatigue, muscle weakness, and difficulty in climbing stairs or rising from a sitting position (from muscle wasting in the pelvis, arms, and legs). Ask about a history of frequent infectious diseases or slow wound healing—suggesting a suppressed immune response. (Remember, however, that Cushing's syndrome may mask infection signs and symptoms.)

Ask the patient if he has a history of peptic ulcers or psychological problems, such as sleep disturbances, mood swings, anxiety, or depression. Also ask about any libido decrease; with a woman, also ask if she's had recent menstrual irregularities.

Adrenal Disorders

A history of spinal-compression fractures, pathologic long-bone fractures, and persistent backache also suggests Cushing's syndrome. These problems may stem from osteoporosis resulting from excess cortisol, which increases calcium resorption from bone and inhibits collagen formation (essential for bone growth). A child with Cushing's syndrome may have stunted linear growth.

Physical examination. Your physical examination involves only general inspection. Begin by noting the patient's appearance. Suspect Cushing's syndrome if he has truncal obesity, cervicodorsal fat (buffalo hump), a moon-shaped face, and/or scrawny arms and legs.

Next, carefully inspect the patient's skin. Protein catabolism from Cushing's syndrome makes the skin fragile, paperlike, and injury-prone. Purplish pink striae wider than 1 cm may appear on the abdomen, buttocks, breasts, and axillae. You may note numerous bruises or mild hematomas, indicating capillary fragility. If your patient has a pituitary or hypothalamic disorder, you may also observe mild skin hyperpigmentation, which results from excessive pituitary ACTH and its subsequent stimulation of melanocytes within the skin.

With a woman, check for signs of masculinization from increased androgen secretion—thinning scalp hair, hirsutism, acne, and clitoral enlargement.

Also measure the patient's blood pressure. Cushing's syndrome may cause mild or moderate hypertension from expanded fluid volume caused by cortisol-induced sodium and water retention.

Diagnostic studies. The doctor will diagnose Cushing's syndrome from laboratory findings. Suggestive results include above-normal serum cortisol levels with no circadian variation and above-normal urinary levels of the steroid metabolites 17-hydroxycorticosteroids (17-OHCS) and 17-ketosteroids (17-KS). The patient may also have elevated red blood cell and granulocyte counts, along with lymphocytopenia and eosinopenia. Secondary Cushing's syndrome causes above-normal serum ACTH levels; primary and iatrogenic Cushing's syndrome lead to below-normal ACTH levels.

Radiologic studies, ultrasonography, angiography, and computerized tomography (CT) scans help identify any adrenal, pituitary, or nonendocrine tumor as the cause of Cushing's syndrome.

Planning

Before determining your nursing care plan, develop the nursing diagnosis by identifying your patient's problem or potential problem, then relating it to its cause. Possible nursing diagnoses for a patient with Cushing's syndrome include:
- skin integrity, impairment of (delayed wound healing); related to protein catabolism
- infection, potential for; related to immunosuppression
- activity intolerance; related to fatigue
- self-concept, disturbances in; related to appearance changes
- knowledge deficit; related to disease process
- fluid volume, alteration in (extracellular volume excess); related to sodium and water retention
- injury, potential for; related to muscle weakness and osteoporosis.

Continued on page 142

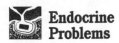
Adrenal Disorders

Sample nursing care plan: Cushing's syndrome

Nursing diagnosis	Expected outcomes
Skin integrity, impairment of (delayed wound healing); related to protein catabolism	The patient will: • show appropriate wound healing. • show he knows how to prevent infection and promote wound healing.
Nursing interventions	**Discharge planning**
• Frequently assess patient's skin for bruising and unhealed lesions. • Use strict aseptic technique when caring for skin lesions or performing invasive procedures. • Monitor wounds for persistent drainage. • Monitor patient's white blood cell count and temperature for signs of infection. • Encourage adequate intake of protein and vitamins A and C to aid wound healing.	• Advise patient to reduce sodium intake to less than 2 g/day and to reduce fluid intake as indicated. • Encourage diet high in protein-rich foods. • Discuss wound prevention and care with patient and his family. • Advise patient to avoid persons with contagious illnesses. • Teach patient about his disease and treatment rationale. • Advise patient when to seek medical care. • Arrange for follow-up care as indicated.

Cushing's syndrome—*continued*

The sample care plan above shows expected outcomes, nursing interventions, and discharge planning for one nursing diagnosis listed on page 141. However, you'll want to tailor each care plan to fit the patient's needs.

Intervention

Treatment of Cushing's syndrome ultimately aims to alleviate the underlying cause. With iatrogenic Cushing's syndrome, the doctor may gradually discontinue steroid therapy if the patient's condition allows. With Cushing's syndrome caused by a pituitary tumor, the doctor may surgically remove the entire pituitary gland or just the tumor, typically using a transsphenoidal approach. (See Chapter 2 for details on transsphenoidal hypophysectomy.) Or, he may order radiation therapy to destroy the pituitary gland (more successful in children).

An adrenocortical tumor necessitates unilateral or bilateral adrenalectomy and postoperative steroid replacement. Temporary steroid replacement usually follows unilateral adrenalectomy (until the remaining atrophied gland resumes function). A patient who's had bilateral adrenalectomy needs lifelong steroid replacement.

For a patient with an inoperable tumor, the doctor may order a drug that inhibits cortisol synthesis—most commonly, aminoglutethimide, metyrapone, or mitotane. (*Note:* Stay alert for signs and symptoms of acute adrenal crisis when administering mitotane—the drug's an extremely potent adrenal inhibitor.) In some cases, he'll order cyproheptadine, an ACTH inhibitor that's particularly useful in secondary Cushing's syndrome.

Signs and symptoms of Cushing's syndrome usually disappear with proper treatment. However, if they don't, the doctor may order spironolactone (Aldactone), a mineralocorticoid antagonist, to relieve hypertension and hypokalemia.

Nursing priorities for a patient with Cushing's syndrome include:
• preventing accidental injury from falls (caused by muscle weakness or pathologic fractures)

Nelson's syndrome

This syndrome arises when a preexisting adrenocorticotropic hormone (ACTH)–secreting pituitary adenoma recurs after bilateral adrenalectomy for Cushing's syndrome. Adrenalectomy removes cortisol's suppressive effects, permitting increased ACTH secretion as well as tumor progression.

Among the most aggressive and rapidly growing pituitary tumors, a Nelson's syndrome tumor leads to hyperpigmentation and signs and symptoms of a growing intrasellar lesion (such as visual field defects or headache). Some patients also experience pituitary apoplexy.

Initial treatment typically involves transfrontal craniotomy or transsphenoidal hypophysectomy. The tumor's large size usually prevents complete resection. In some patients, conventional radiation therapy alone successfully treats Nelson's syndrome. For patients with extrasellar tumor extension, the doctor may order postoperative radiation therapy.

Adrenal Disorders

- preventing infection or detecting it early
- increasing activity tolerance
- promoting effective coping strategies to deal with appearance changes.

Major complications of Cushing's syndrome stem from fluid and electrolyte imbalance. Sodium and water retention may greatly expand intracellular volume, causing hypertension and, in a patient with heart disease, congestive heart failure. Hypokalemia further threatens the heart by potentiating ventricular dysrhythmia. Commonly, the patient feels tired, weak, and irritable. Immunosuppression can predispose the patient to infection, possibly leading to sepsis.

Evaluation

Base your evaluation on the expected outcomes listed on the nursing care plan. To determine if the patient's improved, ask yourself the following questions:

- Does the patient have signs and symptoms of wound infection?
- Have his wounds healed completely and within the expected time?
- Does he know how to prevent wound infection and promote wound healing?
- Does he understand how increased dietary protein and vitamins A and C can help promote wound healing?

The answers to these questions will help you evaluate your patient's status and the effectiveness of his care. Keep in mind that these questions stem from the sample nursing care plan on the opposite page. Your questions may differ.

Adrenocortical insufficiency

Adrenocortical insufficiency includes all disorders involving suppressed adrenocortical function and reduced adrenocortical hormone production. Such disorders may deteriorate into a life-threatening adrenal crisis (see the information under "Complications").

Adrenocortical insufficiency can be primary or secondary. *Primary adrenocortical insufficiency,* also called Addison's disease, reflects an intrinsic pathologic condition affecting both adrenal glands.

Idiopathic adrenal atrophy (usually resulting from an autoimmune disorder) most commonly causes Addison's disease. A relatively rare, chronic disorder, adrenal atrophy may occur spontaneously or insidiously, progressing until only a thin cortical tissue layer surrounds the adrenal medulla. Destructive lesions develop within the adrenal cortex. Usually, signs and symptoms of adrenocortical insufficiency don't appear until the disease destroys nearly 90% of the glands.

Secondary adrenocortical insufficiency reflects reduced ACTH secretion from the anterior pituitary gland, caused by pituitary disease or suppression from exogenous steroid administration.

Because of widespread synthetic steroid use, secondary adrenocortical insufficiency occurs far more commonly than Addison's disease.

Adrenocortical insufficiency: Reviewing the causes

Primary adrenocortical insufficiency (Addison's disease)
Intrinsic adrenal gland destruction, resulting from:
- hemorrhage from anticoagulant therapy
- idiopathic autoimmune atrophy
- histoplasmosis
- infiltrative disease, such as cancer, sarcoidosis, and hemochromatosis
- septicemia (from meningococcal or staphylococcal infection)
- surgical adrenal gland removal
- tuberculosis.

Absent hormone production, resulting from:
- use of inhibitive and cytotoxic drugs (such as metyrapone).

Secondary adrenocortical insufficiency
Pituitary disease, resulting from:
- granulomas (such as leukemia and hemochromatosis)
- idiopathic adrenal gland destruction
- metastatic disease
- pituitary tumor (such as chromophobe adenoma and craniopharyngioma)
- postpartum necrosis (Sheehan's syndrome)
- exogenous stress (such as from trauma or surgery).

Suppression of hypothalamic-pituitary axis, resulting from:
- abrupt steroid therapy withdrawal.

Continued on page 144

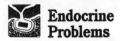
Adrenal Disorders

Adrenocortical insufficiency—*continued*

Adrenocortical insufficiency impairs the patient's stress response by reducing cortisol, aldosterone, and androgen secretion. With primary adrenocortical insufficiency, reduced cortisol levels stimulate ACTH release via a negative feedback mechanism within the hypothalamic-pituitary axis. This ACTH increase has little effect on the destroyed adrenal gland. With secondary adrenocortical insufficiency, ACTH production and secretion decrease, leading to adrenocortical understimulation. Eventually, the adrenal cortex atrophies.

Assessment

As you take the patient's history and perform the physical examination, keep in mind that adrenocortical insufficiency produces clinical changes that reflect decreased or absent glucocorticoid and mineralocorticoid production (see *Adrenocortical insufficiency pathophysiology*).

History. Chief complaints that suggest adrenocortical insufficiency include muscle weakness and fatigue, from reduced cortisol and increased potassium levels. Early in the disease, fatigue may occur only during stressful periods. Also ask about a history of gastrointestinal problems, such as nausea, vomiting, diarrhea, vague abdominal pain, and salt craving. These problems can cause weight loss and exacerbate dehydration, which, in turn, worsens hypotension.

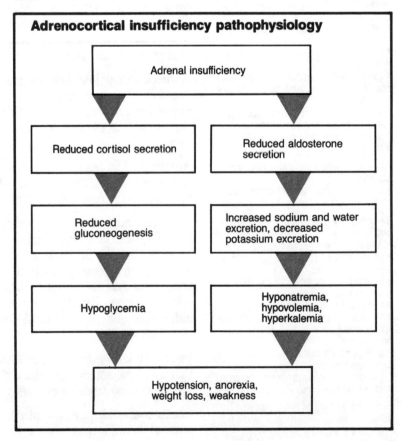

Adrenocortical insufficiency pathophysiology

Adrenal insufficiency

Reduced cortisol secretion

Reduced aldosterone secretion

Reduced gluconeogenesis

Increased sodium and water excretion, decreased potassium excretion

Hypoglycemia

Hyponatremia, hypovolemia, hyperkalemia

Hypotension, anorexia, weight loss, weakness

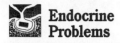
Adrenal Disorders

Because the adrenal cortex proves crucial to the body's stress response, the patient with adrenocortical insufficiency may also report anxiety, restlessness, irritability, and confusion. He may suffer extreme, incapacitating exhaustion from even slight emotional upset or stressful physical conditions, such as mild influenza.

Physical examination. Assess the patient's vital signs for evidence of extracellular volume depletion, sodium loss, and excessive potassium retention (from reduced aldosterone, which inhibits sodium and water reabsorption and potassium excretion by the distal renal tubules). Other common findings include orthostatic hypotension and dehydration. Also check for hyperkalemia signs and symptoms, such as sensory deficits and muscle weakness or paralysis.

Check your patient's skin for hyperpigmentation, a striking but variable feature of the primary disease. Pay particular attention to elbows, knees, and other pressure areas, as well as nipples, palm creases, and scars. The skin may appear darkened—brown or bronze—in both exposed and unexposed areas, resembling a dirty tan (the precise color depends on the patient's ethnic background). Small black freckles may cover the neck, face, and forehead, while bluish black splotches may appear on mucous membranes. Such changes result from increased anterior pituitary ACTH release in response to reduced plasma cortisol levels. Hyperpigmentation also helps differentiate between primary and secondary adrenocortical insufficiency—only the primary disease causes this sign. In a few cases, the patient may have vitiligo, pale patches surrounded by excess pigmentation.

Diagnostic studies. The doctor usually diagnoses adrenocortical insufficiency from laboratory test results. Suggestive findings include below-normal serum cortisol, urinary 17-OHCS, and urinary 17-KS values. Above-normal ACTH values suggest Addison's disease; below-normal ACTH values may mean secondary adrenocortical insufficiency. With a pituitary deficiency, an ACTH stimulation test causes an elevated cortisol level; with a primary adrenal disorder, serum cortisol remains at baseline level. Other laboratory findings that may indicate adrenocortical insufficiency include hyperkalemia; hyponatremia; hypochloremia; fasting hypoglycemia; and above-normal blood urea nitrogen, eosinophil, lymphocyte, and hematocrit values.

An EKG may show hyperkalemia signs, such as sharply peaked T waves and broad QRS complexes. X-rays may reveal decreased heart size (from chronic cardiac output reduction) and adrenal calcifications.

Planning

Before determining your nursing care plan, develop the nursing diagnosis by identifying your patient's problem or potential problem, then relating it to its cause. Possible nursing diagnoses for a patient with primary adrenocortical insufficiency (Addison's disease) include:
• fluid volume, alteration in (extracellular volume deficit); related to aldosterone deficiency

Continued on page 146

Cost-cutting tip

The patient with adrenocortical insufficiency risks *adrenal crisis*. To prevent this emergency and avoid additional hospitalization costs, review the following points with the patient before discharge:
• the pathology and signs and symptoms of chronic adrenocortical insufficiency and the constant risk of adrenal crisis
• proper steroid self-administration, actions and doses of his prescribed medications, and signs and symptoms of excessive or insufficient drug use
• the need to avoid stopping the prescribed steroid or altering the dose without first consulting the doctor
• the need to avoid long fasting periods
• the importance of maintaining a high-carbohydrate, high-protein diet, with a daily sodium intake of up to 8 g (more during diaphoresis)
• the need to call his doctor to have his glucocorticoid dose increased during stressful situations (such as emotional crisis, minor surgery, or infection) or to have his mineralocorticoid dose increased if he sweats profusely for any reason
• the use of relaxation techniques to reduce stress
• the need to intersperse planned activities with rest periods (muscle weakness and decreased hepatic glycogen stores lead to easy fatigue).

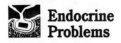
Adrenal Disorders

What to tell a patient taking steroids

If your patient will continue oral steroid therapy at home, review these important points with him before discharge:
• Take the drug only as prescribed. Don't alter the dose or stop taking the drug without consulting your doctor. Sudden withdrawal may precipitate an adrenal crisis.
• Take the drug at mealtimes or with snacks to reduce gastric irritation.
• For alternate-day therapy (common with long-term administration), take twice the usual daily glucocorticoid dose every other morning—preferably before 9 a.m.
• For daily therapy, take a higher dose around 8 a.m. and a lower dose in the afternoon or evening to mimic the body's normal cortisol secretion pattern.
• Establish baseline blood pressure, weight, and sleep patterns, and continually assess them throughout the steroid administration period.
• If ordered, eat a high-potassium, low-sodium diet. Potassium-rich foods include leafy vegetables, avocados, citrus fruits, bananas, and whole grains. Sodium-rich foods that you should avoid include packaged snacks, bouillon, sauces, luncheon meats, canned vegetables, and cheeses.
• Notify the doctor if you have disease exacerbations or undergo severe stress, such as from infection or injury. He may need to adjust your drug dose.
• If you have diabetes mellitus, expect the doctor to closely monitor your blood and urine glucose levels.
• Report any adverse drug effects, such as excessive weight gain, edema, marked muscle weakness, bone pain, hypertension, depression, headache, polyuria, or infection.
• Avoid persons with infectious diseases and notify the doctor if you suspect you have an infection. Also, report delayed wound healing and any vague feelings of sickness (by suppressing the immune system, corticosteroids may mask infections).
• Obtain a medical identification bracelet (such as a Medic Alert bracelet) describing your condition, drug, and dose.
• Visit your doctor regularly.

Sample nursing care plan: Addison's disease

Nursing diagnosis	Expected outcomes
Fluid volume, alteration in (extracellular volume deficit); related to aldosterone deficiency	The patient will: • maintain normal fluid status, as shown by lack of orthostatic hypotension, urinary output of at least 30 ml/hour, and moist mucous membranes. • show he understands disease process, treatment, and ways to prevent exacerbations (adrenal crisis).
Nursing interventions • Assess blood pressure and pulse for orthostatic changes. • Assess intake and output; notify doctor if urine output drops below 30 ml/hour or 240 ml/8-hour shift. • Take daily weights. • Assess skin turgor and mucous membranes for dehydration signs. • Encourage fluid intake of at least 3,000 ml/day. • Instruct patient to increase his salt intake by at least 5 g/day, if indicated. • Warn patient to avoid rising quickly from sitting or reclining position.	**Discharge planning** • Teach patient and family about disease and importance of lifelong management, including the following points: —eating three meals a day —properly self-administering steroids —increasing fluid intake —wearing medical identification, such as a Medic Alert bracelet —carrying an emergency glucocorticoid injection kit —getting regular medical checkups. • Advise patient when to seek medical care. • Arrange for follow-up care if indicated.

Adrenocortical insufficiency—*continued*

• injury, potential for; related to electrolyte imbalance (hyperkalemia, hyponatremia)
• coping, ineffective; related to reduced cortisol levels
• activity intolerance; related to cortisol deficiency and hyperkalemia
• nutrition, alteration in (less than body requirements); related to nausea and/or anorexia
• self-concept, disturbances in; related to appearance changes
• knowledge deficit; related to disease process and treatment.

The sample care plan above shows expected outcomes, nursing interventions, and discharge planning for one nursing diagnosis listed on page 145. However, you'll want to tailor each care plan to the patient's needs.

Intervention

Usually incurable, Addison's disease follows a long, relentless course requiring lifelong hormone replacement. Oral cortisone (Cortone) administration effectively achieves glucocorticoid replacement. The doctor will probably order a dose ranging from 20 to 25 mg in the morning and 10 to 12.5 mg in the afternoon to mimic the body's normal cortisol secretion pattern. For stressful periods, such as minor surgery, dental work, and illness, he'll probably increase the dose. In some cases, he'll order equivalent doses of other glucocorticoids, such as prednisone or prednisolone, instead of cortisone.

If the patient also requires aldosterone replacement, expect the doctor to order the mineralocorticoid fludrocortisone (Florinef) in a dose of 0.1 mg daily or three times a week. A patient with secondary adrenocortical insufficiency doesn't need aldosterone replacement because mineralocorticoid release doesn't depend on ACTH secretion.

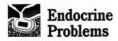
Adrenal Disorders

Advise the patient to salt his food liberally. If indicated, he should increase his salt intake by at least 5 to 8 g per day, particularly if he sweats profusely. Caution him not to fast or omit meals and to eat between-meal and bedtime snacks. Also advise him to eat foods high in carbohydrates and protein.

Instruct the patient to obtain medical identification (such as a Medic Alert bracelet) and an emergency kit containing an injectable glucocorticoid solution (usually 100 mg hydrocortisone) in a sterile syringe ready for injection, along with bystander instructions for use if the patient's found unconscious. Tell him to carry the kit at all times. If indicated, advise him to keep parenteral glucocorticoids at home for I.M. injection during illness, when nausea and vomiting prevent oral steroid administration.

Long-term measures focus on controlling the disease and preventing acute exacerbations. Make sure the patient understands the importance of complying with steroid therapy (for more information on patient guidelines for steroid therapy, see *What to tell a patient taking steroids*).

Complications

Adrenal crisis, the most serious complication of adrenocortical insufficiency, can occur gradually or with catastrophic suddenness. Also known as acute adrenal insufficiency, this potentially lethal condition usually develops in a patient who doesn't respond to hormone replacement therapy or who's undergone marked stress without adequate glucocorticoid replacement. Adrenal crisis can also result from abrupt corticosteroid withdrawal in a patient receiving chronic or high glucocorticoid doses. For this reason, steroid therapy must be withdrawn gradually. Other causes include trauma, burns, hypercoagulability, and hemorrhagic adrenal gland necrosis resulting from bilateral adrenal vein thrombosis. The thrombosis most commonly follows a severe fulminating infection, such as meningococcal or staphylococcal septicemia (Waterhouse-Friderichsen syndrome).

To reverse adrenal crisis, expect to restore the patient's circulating cortisol and fluid volume by rapidly infusing dextrose 5% in normal saline solution (extracellular volume may drop as much as 20%). Check the patient's vital signs and urine output frequently, and monitor his EKG for serious dysrhythmias. As ordered, also monitor his hemodynamic parameters (central venous or pulmonary capillary wedge pressure) and check regularly for pulmonary crackles, edema, jugular vein distention, and extra heart sounds to help assess his volume status.

As ordered, administer cortisol (hydrocortisone [Solu-Cortef]) I.V. every 6 hours until acute signs and symptoms subside. Although cortisol doesn't totally replace aldosterone, it proves adequate if given with sufficient saline solution. Hyperkalemia usually responds rapidly to cortisol and saline solution administration and typically warrants no other therapy. (*Caution:* Don't give methylprednisolone [Solu-Medrol], because this drug lacks hydrocortisone's mineralocorticoid effects.)

Continued on page 148

Adrenal crisis: A quick review

What to assess for:
- Headache, confusion, dizziness, restlessness, apathy
- Pallor
- Increased respiratory rate
- Fatigue, muscle weakness
- Hypoglycemia
- Nausea, vomiting, diarrhea, abdominal cramps, weight loss, appetite loss
- Dehydration, reduced urinary output
- Hyperkalemia
- Increased pulse rate
- Hypotension

How to intervene:
- Maintain patent airway and breathing.
- Maintain circulation by giving I.V. fluids, such as dextrose 5% in normal saline solution.
- Replace glucocorticoids by giving I.V. hydrocortisone (Solu-Cortef).

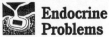
Adrenal Disorders

Adrenocortical insufficiency—*continued*

As you care for the patient with adrenal crisis, be aware that illness-induced anxiety can exacerbate his condition. To help reduce anxiety, maintain a calm approach and explain all nursing procedures.

Evaluation

Base your evaluation on the expected outcomes listed on the nursing care plan. To determine if your patient's improved, ask yourself the following questions:

• Can the patient maintain adequate fluid volume, as shown by lack of orthostatic hypotension, urinary output of at least 30 ml/hr, and moist mucous membranes?
• Does he understand his disease and its treatment?
• Does he know how to prevent dehydration?
• Does he know when to seek medical attention?

The answers to these questions will help you evaluate your patient's status and the effectiveness of his care. Keep in mind that these questions stem from the sample nursing care plan on page 146. Your questions may differ.

Multiple endocrine neoplasia syndromes

Familial disorders, multiple endocrine neoplasia (MEN) syndromes involve concurrent hyperplasia, adenomas, or cancerous tumors in two or more endocrine glands. These three distinct MEN patterns have been identified.

MEN type I
(Wermer's syndrome)
Gland and neoplastic changes:
• Pancreatic islet cell tumor
• Parathyroid hyperplasia or adenoma
• Pituitary tumor

Associated abnormalities:
• Lipomas
• Peptic ulcer
• Zollinger-Ellison syndrome

MEN type II
(Sipple's syndrome)
Gland and neoplastic changes:
• Parathyroid hyperplasia or adenoma
• Pheochromocytoma
• Thyroidal medullary cancer

Associated abnormalities:
• Cushing's syndrome
• Diarrhea

MEN type III
(also known as type IIb)
Gland and neoplastic changes:
• Pheochromocytoma
• Thyroidal medullary cancer

Associated abnormalities:
• Lip enlargement
• Marfanoid physique
• Neuromas

Assessment findings and intervention depend on the affected glands and associated disorders.

Pheochromocytoma

A rare, usually benign chromaffin cell tumor, pheochromocytoma typically arises within the medulla of one or both adrenal glands. The disorder results in hypersecretion of epinephrine and/or norepinephrine (and, in some cases, also dopamine). These encapsulated, highly vascular tumors may also appear outside the adrenal gland, within the sympathetic ganglia of the abdomen, chest, and cervical area (extra-adrenal pheochromocytomas, or paragangliomas). Tumors appear more commonly in the right adrenal gland than in the left. Epinephrine overproduction occurs only with adrenal pheochromocytoma, whereas norepinephrine overproduction can occur with either an adrenal or an extra-adrenal tumor. Middle-aged women have an increased risk for pheochromocytoma.

Pheochromocytoma can also occur in conjunction with thyroidal medullary cancer and hyperparathyroidism—a combined disease entity known as multiple endocrine neoplasia type II (MEN type II, or Sipple's syndrome). See *Multiple endocrine neoplasia syndromes* for details.

Assessment

Because pheochromocytoma produces and secretes excessive catecholamines into the bloodstream, the patient will suffer effects such as those in an exaggerated flight or fight reaction. The disorder's hallmark—high blood pressure—typically resembles essential hypertension. Blood pressure may fluctuate, reaching 200/150 mm Hg or even higher. With persistent hypertension, you may detect signs of end-organ damage, such as cerebrovascular accident, retinopathy, heart disease, or kidney damage. Obtain standing, sitting, and lying blood pressure measurements. Because chronically excessive catecholamine levels may eventually impair the postural reflexes that maintain upright blood pressure, the patient may have

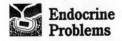
Adrenal Disorders

orthostatic hypotension. Ask him if he gets dizzy, light-headed, or faint, particularly when assuming an upright position.

A paroxysm, or attack—perhaps the most classic finding—occurs if the tumor releases catecholamines sporadically. In a typical attack, the patient feels unusual chest sensations, triggering deeper breathing. A pounding heartbeat follows, resulting from increased cardiac output (controlled by $beta_1$-receptors). Pounding spreads throughout the trunk and to the head, causing headache or throbbing. Moist, cool hands and feet and facial pallor result from enhanced alpha-receptor–mediated peripheral vasoconstriction. Increased cardiac output and vasoconstriction lead to pronounced hypertension with release of excess catecholamines. Elevated body temperature or flushing, causing reflex sweating, may result from diminished heat loss and heightened metabolism. Sweating may be profuse and typically follows cardiovascular effects. Blood glucose levels rise from elevated glycolysis and alpha-receptor–mediated insulin inhibition.

During all but the mildest attack, the patient feels extremely anxious. With a prolonged or severe attack, he may have vomiting, nausea, visual disturbances, chest or abdominal pain, paresthesias, and seizures. Afterward, he'll probably feel exhausted.

Attacks may occur as frequently as several times daily or as seldom as once a year. They may last from a few seconds to several hours. Ask the patient if anything seems to bring on the attack. Although symptoms sometimes arise spontaneously, they may result from such stimuli as exercise, heavy lifting, emotional distress, exposure to cold, food or alcohol intake, bladder distention, defecation, sexual intercourse, or abdominal palpation. Instruct the patient to notify the doctor when the attack begins so that blood pressure can be measured.

Diagnostic studies. To diagnose pheochromocytoma, the doctor must rule out conditions that cause similar signs and symptoms—hyperthyroidism, menopause, essential hypertension, angina pectoris, transient ischemic attacks, acute anxiety, and interactions between monoamine oxidase inhibitors and tyramine-rich foods (such as aged cheese).

Expect him to order various laboratory tests. Suggestive findings include an above-normal fasting blood glucose level—probably from catecholamines' antagonistic effects on insulin as well as from increased hepatic glucose output. Rarely extreme, the resulting hyperglycemia almost never requires specific treatment. The patient may also have an above-normal hematocrit value, reflecting diminished plasma volume or, perhaps, catecholamines' erythropoietin-stimulating effect.

For a definitive diagnosis, the doctor will order 24-hour urine collection of catecholamines and their metabolites. Urinary metanephrine, a catecholamine metabolite, gives more reliable results than urinary vanillylmandelic acid, an epinephrine metabolite.

EKG changes may also suggest pheochromocytoma. Such changes reflect left ventricular strain from high blood pressure and cate-

Continued on page 150

Adrenal Disorders

Pheochromocytoma—*continued*

cholamine-induced beta-adrenergic stimulation. Expect ST-segment and/or T-wave changes, prominent U waves, tachycardia or bradycardia, and ventricular dysrhythmias. Signs of left ventricular enlargement may also appear.

CT scans help locate the tumor. Radionuclide imaging and selective venographic sampling angiography may also prove useful. However, these tests may precipitate a hypertensive crisis. To avoid this risk, the doctor will order pretest drug therapy to establish effective adrenergic blockade.

Planning

Before determining your nursing care plan, develop the nursing diagnosis by identifying your patient's problem or potential problem, then relating it to its cause. Possible nursing diagnoses for a patient with pheochromocytoma include:
• tissue perfusion, alteration in; related to vasopressive effects of catecholamine excess
• anxiety; related to catecholamine excess
• comfort, alteration in (pain); related to paroxysmal attack
• knowledge deficit; related to disease process or treatment
• fear; related to surgery.

The sample care plan below shows expected outcomes, nursing interventions, and discharge planning for one nursing diagnosis listed above. However, you'll want to tailor each care plan to the patient's needs.

Intervention

In most cases, the doctor will surgically remove the pheochromocytoma (see *Adrenalectomy: Reducing postoperative risks*). Before sur-

Continued on page 152

Sample nursing care plan: Pheochromocytoma

Nursing diagnosis	Expected outcomes
Tissue perfusion, alteration in; related to vasopressive effects of catecholamine excess	The patient will: • maintain adequate vital-organ perfusion, as shown by normal neurologic, renal, and cardiac function. • maintain adequate peripheral circulation. • have fewer paroxysmal attacks.

Nursing interventions	Discharge planning
• Assess blood pressure and pulse; check for orthostatic changes. • Assess peripheral circulation (capillary refill time, skin color, and peripheral pulses) for signs of adequate perfusion. • Assess neurologic status and renal and cardiac function for signs of adequate tissue perfusion. • Monitor any paroxysmal attacks and identify their potential triggers (for example, smoking, exposure to cold, constipation, extreme emotions, and heavy lifting). • Discuss with patient methods that help prevent paroxysmal attacks. • Use relaxation techniques to reduce patient's anxiety.	• Teach patient about disease and prescribed treatment (such as drugs or surgery). • Discuss with patient possible triggers for paroxysmal attacks and ways to avoid them. • Teach patient how to use relaxation techniques. • Teach patient and family how to measure blood pressure, and encourage frequent blood pressure monitoring. • Advise patient when to seek medical assistance. • Arrange for follow-up care if indicated.

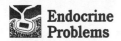

Adrenal Disorders

Adrenalectomy: Reducing postoperative risks

Various adrenal disorders warrant adrenalectomy—removal of one or both adrenal glands. To remove the right adrenal gland, the surgeon moves the colon's hepatic flexure downward and moves the duodenum medially. After retracting the right kidney, he identifies the right adrenal gland in the perinephric fat (see illustration below). To locate the left adrenal gland, he moves the colon's left portion downward, separates the splenocolic ligament, and moves the spleen and pancreas.

In both procedures, the surgeon uses silver clips to control blood vessels. He must be especially careful when securing the right adrenal vein—this short, wide vessel empties directly into the vena cava.

Because the adrenal glands help maintain homeostasis and facilitate the body's stress response, adrenalectomy carries a high risk of postoperative complications. Pheochromocytoma excision proves particularly delicate because it can lead to a transient increase in circulating adrenal hormone and catecholamine levels. Follow the guidelines below to help minimize postoperative problems.

Preoperative care. To help the patient withstand surgery and improve postoperative wound healing, administer parenteral cortisol (usually hydrocortisone), as ordered, and provide a diet high in protein and vitamins. To correct any electrolyte imbalances, make sure the patient receives appropriate supplements. For example, a patient with adrenocortical hyperfunction should receive potassium supplements as well as potassium-rich foods. Explain the surgical procedure and expected postoperative measures, such as I.V. infusions, hemodynamic monitoring, and nasogastric suctioning. Teach the patient how to perform coughing and deep breathing to prevent postoperative infection.

Postoperative care. If your patient's had bilateral adrenalectomy, he'll lack adrenocortical hormones and adrenal medullary catecholamines. To prevent adrenal crisis, monitor him carefully and give fluids, electrolytes, and corticosteroids, as ordered.

Postoperative blood pressure and fluid and electrolyte levels may fluctuate widely, especially in the first 48 hours. During and after surgery, monitor the patient's EKG and arterial, central venous, and (if indicated) pulmonary capillary wedge pressures to evaluate his hemodynamic status.

Expect to give I.V. replacement glucocorticoids until the patient can tolerate oral doses. The doctor may order fluid replacement with dextrose 5% in water and normal saline solution, as well as vasopressors to prevent hypovolemic shock.

Your ongoing assessment will help evaluate the patient's response to therapy. Carefully record his vital signs, intake, and output. Stay alert for signs and symptoms of adrenocortical insufficiency—lethargy, apathy, nausea, hypoglycemia, hyponatremia, and hyperkalemia—and report them at once.

Immediately after surgery, withhold foods and fluids. Introduce oral intake gradually, according to the patient's tolerance. Because his condition may rule out prolonged fasting, he'll probably require I.V. calorie supplements. After he begins eating, make sure he doesn't miss any meals, and offer him between-meal snacks. Stay alert for hypoglycemia signs and symptoms. To reduce anxiety, anticipate stressful situations and try to prevent them. Provide for sufficient rest periods and comfort measures.

To promote wound healing, scrupulously monitor the patient's temperature and wound drainage, and use strict aseptic technique when changing his dressings. Make sure he splints his wound during coughing or turning to reduce pressure on the wound. Watch closely for wound dehiscence and evisceration.

Before discharge, discuss the importance of taking cortisol supplements regularly to treat adrenocortical insufficiency.

Transabdominal approach to right adrenal gland

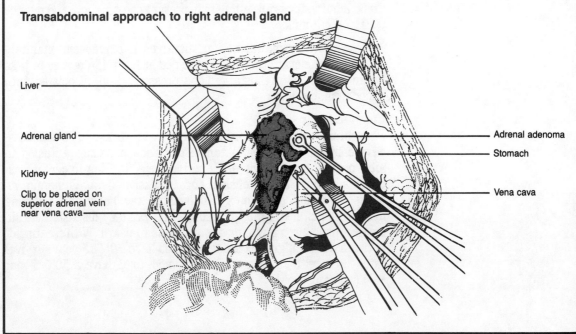

Liver

Adrenal gland

Kidney

Clip to be placed on superior adrenal vein near vena cava

Adrenal adenoma

Stomach

Vena cava

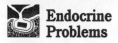
Adrenal Disorders

Pheochromocytoma—*continued*

gery, however, he'll order drugs to reverse the effects of excessive adrenergic stimulation. Adrenergic blocking agents include alpha-adrenergic blockers (most commonly, phenoxybenzamine [Dibenzyline]), the preferred drugs; and selective alpha-antagonists, such as prazosin (Minipress). The patient must take the prescribed drug for 2 weeks.

Beta-adrenergic blocking agents, such as propranolol, prove useful adjuncts in treating pheochromocytoma. The doctor may order these drugs after establishing alpha-adrenergic blockade. Propranolol particularly helps control catecholamine-induced dysrhythmias, angina, and sweating.

Preoperative management also includes careful plasma volume reexpansion—usually achieved with liberal salt intake. During surgery, the patient will probably receive I.V. infusions of the alpha-adrenergic blocker phentolamine (Regitine) to prevent hypertensive crisis from anesthesia induction and tumor manipulation; and nitroprusside (a potent vasodilator) to help manage hypertensive crisis. After tumor removal, blood pressure may drop, which necessitates volume expansion with whole blood, plasma, or fluids. A benign tumor may recur after surgery.

For a patient who doesn't qualify for surgery or doesn't respond to conventional therapy, the doctor may order a drug that inhibits catecholamine synthesis, such as metyrosine (Demser). Such drugs inhibit hydroxylase, an enzyme that promotes norepinephrine synthesis. Warn the patient to avoid drugs that potentiate catecholamine's effects and may lead to fatal paroxysmal crisis. Such drugs include opiates, histamine, glucagon, metoclopramide, guanethidine, tricyclic antidepressants, and droperidol. Also tell him to avoid over-the-counter cold medications and decongestants, unless the doctor approves.

Try to identify potential triggers for paroxysmal attacks, and, if possible, eliminate them. For example, keep room temperature moderate, administer stool softeners to prevent constipation, and provide a calm environment.

During a paroxysmal attack or sustained hypertension, maintain bed rest and elevate the head of the bed at least 45 degrees to take advantage of the orthostatic blood pressure drop associated with pheochromocytoma.

Complications

Pheochromocytoma complications can have serious consequences. Severe hypotension, for instance, can reduce tissue perfusion to vital organs, such as the brain and kidneys, leading to cerebrovascular accident. Hypertension and excessive beta-adrenergic responses to catecholamines can overtax the heart, precipitating dysrhythmias, heart failure, and coronary artery disease. Left untreated, pheochromocytoma always leads to death. With treatment, patients with benign pheochromocytoma have a 95% 5-year survival rate; those with cancerous pheochromocytoma have a 50% 5-year survival rate.

Adrenal Disorders

Evaluation

Base your evaluation on the expected outcomes listed on the nursing care plan. To determine if your patient's improved, ask yourself the following questions:
- Has the patient's blood pressure stabilized?
- Does he have fewer paroxysmal attacks?
- Does he have adequate tissue perfusion?
- Does he understand the disease process and treatment goals?
- Does he know what triggers his paroxysmal attacks and how he can avoid or minimize these triggers?

The answers to these questions will help you evaluate your patient's status and the effectiveness of his care. Keep in mind that these questions stem from the sample nursing care plan on page 150. Your questions may differ.

Other adrenal gland disorders

Aldosteronism

Aldosteronism develops from excessive secretion of mineralocorticoids, primarily aldosterone. The disorder can be primary or secondary. *Primary aldosteronism* (also called Conn's syndrome) results from intrinsic adrenocortical disease—usually a benign aldosterone-producing adenoma. *Secondary aldosteronism* results from a pathologic condition outside the adrenal cortex—most commonly, excess renin-angiotensin system stimulation. Such stimulation can occur with any condition that reduces circulating blood volume or renal blood flow, for example, pregnancy, hypovolemia, congestive heart failure, chronic renal failure, renal artery stenosis, Bartter's syndrome, cirrhosis, Wilms' tumor, or oral contraceptive use. (*Note:* Excessive ingestion of black licorice can cause effects mimicking aldosteronism.)

Assessment. Signs and symptoms of aldosteronism reflect aldosterone's exaggerated renal effects. For example, aldosterone-induced renal sodium and water retention can greatly expand blood volume, leading to marked hypertension. The patient may complain of headaches or visual disturbances. Surprisingly, edema rarely occurs with primary aldosteronism but commonly accompanies secondary aldosteronism. Also check for signs and symptoms of congestive heart failure, especially in a patient with a known cardiac disorder.

Hypokalemia occurs as aldosterone stimulates sodium-potassium exchange in the kidney's distal tubules. This leads to urinary potassium depletion, which, in turn, causes neuromuscular alterations and subsequent muscle weakness and cardiac dysrhythmias. Check for signs and symptoms of metabolic alkalosis, such as lip or finger tingling and paresthesia—chronic hypokalemia potentiates hydrogen ion loss via urine. Also check for increased urinary output. This may arise as prolonged hypokalemia reduces distal tubule sensitivity to antidiuretic hormone, thus precipitating renal diabetes insipidus and excessive dilute urine output (see *Primary aldosteronism: Reviewing the pathophysiology,* page 154, for details).

The doctor usually diagnoses aldosteronism from laboratory tests and EKG results. Suspect aldosteronism if findings reveal spontaneous hypokalemia (in a patient with hypertension) and above-

Continued on page 154

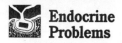
Adrenal Disorders

Congenital adrenal hyperplasia

The most common adrenal disorder in infants and children, congenital adrenal hyperplasia, (CAH) results from a defect in at least six enzymes involved in cortisol synthesis. Because these enzymes don't manufacture adequate cortisol, circulating cortisol levels drop. This, in turn, stimulates adrenocorticotropic hormone (ACTH) secretion by the anterior pituitary gland, causing adrenal hyperplasia.

Deficient 21-hydroxylase (an autosomal recessive trait) accounts for about 95% of CAH cases. Although this enzyme's essential for cortisol and aldosterone synthesis, it doesn't contribute to androgen and estrogen synthesis. Consequently, its deficiency decreases cortisol and aldosterone biosynthesis and increases ACTH secretion. This leads to increased testosterone production. Because androgen synthesis doesn't require 21-hydroxylase, ACTH-induced adrenal hyperplasia enhances androgen production. (Remember—most adrenal androgens are testosterone precursors.)

Assessment. Signs and symptoms of CAH reflect testosterone overproduction (leading to virilization) and cortisol and aldosterone underproduction (leading to sodium wasting, volume depletion, and hypotension). Thus, a female newborn with CAH may have ambiguous genitalia—an enlarged clitoris and fused labia, but a normal genital tract and gonads. As she grows, she'll develop masculinization signs, such as early pubic and axillary hair, facial hair, a deep voice, and acne. She'll also have markedly delayed or absent breast development or menses.

The male newborn with CAH usually has no apparent abnormality. However, he'll later show signs of accelerated prepubertal virilization and precocious puberty, including an enlarged penis, abundant pubic and axillary hair, and a deep voice. Both girls and boys with CAH appear tall for their age from rapid muscle and bone growth. However, excessive androgen levels eventually hasten epiphyseal closure, producing abnormally short adult stature.

Continued

Primary aldosteronism: Reviewing the pathophysiology

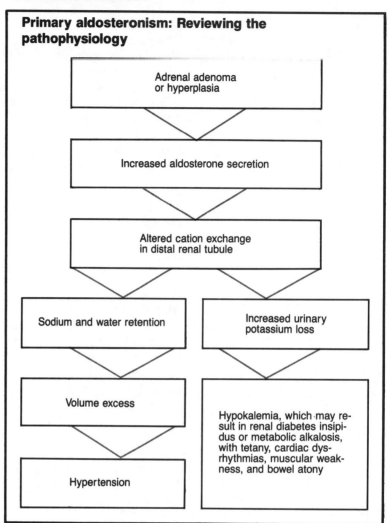

Other adrenal gland disorders—*continued*

normal serum aldosterone and urinary potassium levels (urinary potassium usually exceeds 30 mEq/liter). With renal diabetes insipidus, expect an above-normal serum sodium level and below-normal urine specific gravity. Serum renin levels can help differentiate between primary and secondary aldosteronism—these levels drop abnormally in the former and rise abnormally in the latter. Serum bicarbonate levels may rise abnormally from distal tubule hydrogen and potassium ion loss.

Once the doctor identifies primary aldosteronism, he must further distinguish the cause as adrenal adenoma or bilateral adrenal hyperplasia (the latter's less responsive to surgery). Radionuclide adrenal scans help visualize underlying pathologic changes. However, the doctor may perform adrenal vein catheterization for aldosterone measurement. Elevated venous aldosterone in a single adrenal gland indicates adrenal adenoma; elevation in both glands indicates bilateral hyperplasia.

Other useful diagnostic evidence includes EKG signs of hypokalemia (such as U waves, flattened T waves, and ventricular dysrhythmias) and left ventricular hypertrophy from chronic hypertension, as shown on an EKG or X-ray.

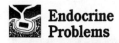
Adrenal Disorders

Continued

Congenital adrenal hyperplasia
Continued

In mild CAH, aldosterone levels remain sufficient to maintain blood pressure and sodium balance. With more severely impaired aldosterone synthesis (called salt-wasting CAH), sodium wasting, volume depletion, and excessive potassium retention develop. In this case, external genitalia appear even more ambiguous. A female newborn may be assigned the wrong sex identification. Without prompt treatment, this CAH form can lead to severe dehydration and hyperkalemia, possibly precipitating cardiovascular collapse.

The doctor will diagnose CAH from the physical examination and laboratory findings. Serum aldosterone and cortisol levels may appear normal or below normal, with above-normal circulating 17-hydroxyprogesterone levels. Urinary 17-ketosteroids and pregnanetriol levels may increase above normal. Urinary 17-hydroxycorticosteroids may be normal or below normal. In salt-wasting CAH, findings also include hyponatremia, hyperkalemia, hypochloremia, and increased hematocrit (hemoconcentration). Ultrasound, computed tomography scans, and other imaging methods can differentiate between CAH and an adrenal gland or ovarian tumor.

Intervention. The patient will require daily cortisol administration to inhibit excessive pituitary ACTH production. A newborn will probably receive parenteral cortisone doses for at least 18 months, then lifelong oral doses. The patient with salt-wasting CAH must also take aldosterone supplements (usually desoxycorticosterone). Advise this patient (or his parents) to increase his dietary sodium intake and restrict his potassium intake.

To determine the sex of a newborn with CAH, the doctor will order sex chromatin and karyotype studies. Reconstructive surgery, usually performed when the patient's between ages 1 and 3, corrects labial fusion and other genital anomalies. Provide emotional support to the parents, and refer them to counseling to help them relate to their child.

Intervention. The doctor will order measures that treat the disease's underlying cause, help reduce blood pressure, and correct hypokalemia. Primary aldosteronism from an adrenal tumor usually necessitates total or partial adrenalectomy. However, blood pressure and renin levels may remain elevated for a month or more postoperatively.

Medical management of primary aldosteronism involves administration of spironolactone, an aldosterone-antagonizing diuretic. Other diuretics may worsen the patient's condition by reducing potassium levels and precipitating serious cardiac dysrhythmias. Potassium supplements serve as important therapeutic adjuncts. (*Note:* If you're administering potassium supplements containing bicarbonate [for example, "fizzies"], be aware that potassium and hydrogen ions compete for absorption in the distal tubules. Therefore, the patient may need to take more supplements to obtain the desired effects.) Expect the doctor to order sodium restriction—as less sodium enters the distal tubules, potassium secretion decreases.

Complications. Aldosteronism can lead to hypertension and hypokalemia, possibly causing neurologic impairment, congestive heart failure, lethal cardiac dysrhythmias, and profound muscle weakness.

Adrenogenital syndrome

This syndrome stems from adrenal androgen overproduction resulting from a tumor or adrenocortical hyperplasia. It may be acquired (adrenal virilism) or congenital (congenital adrenal hyperplasia [CAH]).

A relatively rare disorder, adrenal virilism usually occurs secondary to a benign or cancerous adrenocortical tumor. It affects twice as many women as men. CAH can occur at any age; however, it's the most common adrenal disorder of infants and children.

Whatever the cause, adrenogenital syndrome results in virilization and masculinization. Androgens ultimately undergo conversion to testosterone, an extremely potent hormone that can produce noticeable body changes even when present in small amounts.

Assessment. Adrenogenital syndrome's clinical effects depend on the disorder's cause and the patient's age and sex. A prepubescent boy may have an adult-sized penis, prostate development, and hirsutism. However, despite these premature secondary sex characteristics, the testes fail to mature. In a man, you may have trouble detecting signs of abnormal virilization because of concurrent testicular testosterone production.

In a prepubescent girl, you'll probably notice pubic hair and an enlarged clitoris; in a pubescent girl, absent breast development and delayed menses onset. In a woman, the disorder causes extreme hirsutism with dense hair distribution on the trunk, arms, and legs and pubic hair extension to the navel. You may also observe temporal baldness, acne, a deep voice, an enlarged clitoris, uterine atrophy, amenorrhea, and breast atrophy.

Laboratory findings include above-normal serum testosterone and urinary 17-KS levels (the latter remain high despite dexamethasone administration).

Continued on page 156

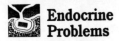
Adrenal Disorders

Other adrenal gland disorders—*continued*

Intervention. For the patient with acquired adrenogenital syndrome, treatment consists of prompt surgical tumor removal. If the tumor has spread to other sites, the doctor will order a neoplastic drug such as mitotane, with or without local radiation therapy. Preoperatively, the patient may require glucocorticoid administration. To detect tumor recurrence, the patient should have periodic follow-up tests. If necessary, refer him and his family for psychological counseling to help them cope with emotional trauma caused by ambiguous sexual characteristics.

Nursing goals include improving the patient's self-image, providing emotional support to him and his family, and encouraging mutual support among family members.

Self-Test

1. Adrenocortical hormones include all of the following except:
a. androgens   b. glucocorticoids   c. mineralocorticoids
d. catecholamines

2. Adrenocortical insufficiency also goes by the name:
a. Cushing's syndrome   b. Cushing's disease   c. Addison's disease   d. pheochromocytoma

3. If your patient's taking steroids, advise him to do all of the following except:
a. alter the dose or stop taking the medication if he becomes sick
b. take the highest dose in the morning   c. take the medication with meals or a snack   d. avoid persons with infectious diseases

4. If your patient has an adrenal crisis, expect to do all of the following except:
a. maintain a patent airway and breathing   b. maintain circulation with rapid I.V. fluid replacement   c. give Solu-Cortef I.V.
d. give Solu-Medrol I.V.

5. Which of the following factors doesn't regulate adrenocorticotropic hormone secretion?
a. circulating cortisol levels   b. adrenal medulla function
c. stress   d. circadian rhythms

6. Which of the following is a classic sign of pheochromocytoma?
a. high blood pressure   b. generalized or localized hyperpigmentation   c. truncal obesity   d. weight loss

Answers (page number shows where answer appears in text)
1. **d** (page 131)   2. **c** (page 143)   3. **a** (page 146)   4. **d** (page 147)   5. **b** (page 130)   6. **a** (page 148)

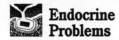

Selected References

Books

Bloodworth, J.M., Jr., ed. *Endocrine Pathology: General and Surgical,* 2nd ed. Baltimore: Williams & Wilkins Co., 1982.

DeGroot, Leslie J., et al. *The Thyroid and Its Diseases,* 5th ed. New York: John Wiley & Sons, 1984.

Ellenberg, Max, and Rifkin, Harold, eds. *Diabetes Mellitus: Theory and Practice,* 3rd ed. New Hyde Park, N.Y.: Medical Examination Publishing Co., 1983.

Felig, Philip, et al. *Endocrinology and Metabolism.* New York: McGraw-Hill Book Co., 1981.

Fischbach, Frances. *A Manual of Laboratory Diagnostic Tests,* 2nd ed. Philadelphia: J.B. Lippincott Co., 1984.

Greenspan, F., and Forsham, P. *Basic and Clinical Endocrinology.* Los Altos, Calif.: Lange Medical Pubs., 1983.

Guyton, Arthur C. *Human Physiology and Mechanisms of Disease,* 3rd ed. Philadelphia: W.B. Saunders Co., 1982.

Hershman, J.M., ed. *Endocrine Pathophysiology: A Patient-Oriented Approach.* Philadelphia: Lea & Febiger, 1982.

Jubiz, William. *Endocrinology: A Logical Approach for Clinicians,* 2nd ed. New York: McGraw-Hill Book Co., 1985.

Krieger, Dorothy T., and Bardin, C. Wayne. *Current Therapy in Endocrinology, 1983-1984.* St. Louis: C.V. Mosby Co., 1983.

Lewis, J.G. *The Endocrine System,* 2nd ed. New York: Churchill Livingstone, 1984.

Marble, A., et al., eds. *Joslin's Diabetes Mellitus,* 12th ed. Philadelphia: Lea & Febiger, 1985.

Marsden, P., and McCullagh, A.G. *Endocrinology.* Littleton, Mass.: PSG Publishing Co., 1985.

Ravel, Richard. *Clinical Laboratory Medicine: Clinical Application of Laboratory Data,* 4th ed. Chicago: Year Book Medical Pubs., 1984.

Rifkin, Harold, ed. *The Physician's Guide to Type II Diabetes (NIDDM).* New York: American Diabetes Association, 1984.

Streck, William F., and Lockwood, Dean H., eds. *Endocrine Diagnosis: Clinical and Laboratory Approach.* Boston: Little, Brown & Co., 1983.

Thompson, June M., et al. *Clinical Nursing.* St. Louis: C.V. Mosby Co., 1986.

Tilkian, Sarko M., and Tilkian, Ara G. *Clinical Implications of Laboratory Tests,* 3rd ed. St. Louis: C.V. Mosby Co., 1983.

Wiener, M.B., and Pepper, G.A. *Clinical Pharmacology and Therapeutics in Nursing,* 2nd ed. New York: McGraw-Hill Book Co., 1985.

Williams, Robert H. *Textbook of Endocrinology,* 6th ed. Philadelphia: W.B. Saunders Co., 1981.

Wilson, J.S., and Foster, D.W. *Williams' Textbook of Endocrinology,* 7th ed. Philadelphia: W.B. Saunders Co., 1985.

Wyngaarden, James B., and Smith, Lloyd H. *Cecil Textbook of Medicine,* 17th ed. Philadelphia: W.B. Saunders Co., 1985.

Periodicals

Evangelisti, Judith, and Thorpe, Constance. "Thyroid Storm—A Nursing Crisis," *Heart & Lung* 12(2):184-93, March 1983.

Larson, C.A. "The Critical Path of Acute Adrenocortical Insufficiency," *Nursing84* 14(10):66-69, October 1984.

Martyn, Pamela. "If You Guessed Cardiovascular Disease, Guess Again," *American Journal of Nursing* 82(8):1239, August 1982.

Ravel, Richard. "Problems in Thyroid Testing," *Emergency Medicine* 14:194-96, May 30, 1982.

Rice, Vee. "Magnesium, Calcium, and Phosphate Imbalances: Their Clinical Significance," *Critical Care Nurse* 3(3), May/June 1983.

Robertson, Carolyn. "Clear the Exercise Hurdles for Your Diabetic Patient," *Nursing84* 14(10):58-63, October 1984.

Robinson, A.G. "Acute Adrenal Insufficiency: Addisonian Crisis," *Topics in Emergency Medicine* 5(4):40-44, January 1984.

Safran, Marjorie, and Braverman, Lewis. "Thyrotoxicosis and Graves' Disease," *Hospital Practice* 20(3A):32-42, 46-49, March 30, 1985.

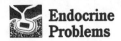
Index

A

Accu-Chek bG, 112i
Acetohexamide, 108, 109
Acromegaly, 32, 34i
ACTH. *See* Adrenocorticotropic hormone.
ACTH stimulation test, 138
Addison's disease. *See* Adrenocortical insufficiency.
Adenohypophysis, 4i, 17, 18i
Adenoma, 30
    classification, 31
ADH. *See* Antidiuretic hormone.
Adrenal crisis, 147-148
Adrenal disorders, 130-156
Adrenalectomy, 151i
Adrenal glands, anatomy of, 4-5i, 130, 131i
Adrenal hormones, 130, 132t
Adrenal virilism, 155-156
Adrenocortical functioning, 130, 133
Adrenocortical insufficiency, 143-148
    assessment, 144-145
    care plan, 146
    intervention, 146-147
    pathophysiology, 144
Adrenocorticotropic hormone, 19, 20t
    deficiency, 33
    excess, 32
    levels, measurement of, 28
Adrenomedullary functioning, 133-134
Aldosterone, 130, 132t, 133
Aldosteronism, 153-155
Alimentary hypoglycemia, 123-124, 125
Alpha-/beta-adrenergic stimulation, 134, 134t
Amines, 6
Aminoglutethimide, 142
Anaplastic carcinoma, 63
Androgenital syndrome, 155-156
Androgens, 130, 132t
Anticholinergics, 128
Antidiuretic hormone, 20-21, 20t
    levels, measurement of, 29
Apoplexy, pituitary, 34
Atriopeptin, 6
Autoimmune hypoglycemia, 125
Autoimmunity, as predisposing factor in diabetes mellitus, 97

B

Biostater Glucose Controller, 107i
Blood chemistry findings in endocrine disorders, 14t
Blood glucose regulation, 91-92
Blood glucose self-monitoring, 111, 112i, 113
Bone mineralization, 70
Bone resorption, 70

C

Calcitonin, 48, 49i, 52, 52t, 70t, 71-72
    levels, measurement of, 57
    role of, in calcium level reduction, 82
Calcitonin secretion test, 74
Calcium, 72-73
    levels, drugs to decrease, 82
    -phosphate metabolism, role of PTH in, 70-71
Calcium supplements, parenteral, 88

Carbamazepine, 42
Carbohydrate metabolism, 91-92
Carbon dioxide, as parahormone, 7
Catecholamine-induced effects, 134t
Chemstrip bG, 112i
Chlorpropamide, 42, 108, 109
Cholecystokinin, as parahormone, 7
Chvostek's sign, 85i
Clinitest, 112i
Clofibrate, 42
Clomid stimulation test, 28
Clomiphene stimulation test, 28
Congenital adrenal hyperplasia, 154-155
Corticosteroids, 61, 62, 133
Corticotropin, 19, 20t
Cortisol, 130, 132t
Cortisone glucose tolerance, 94
Coupling, iodinated precursor, 48
Craniopharyngiomas, 31
Cretinism, 64
Cushing's disease, 32
    vs. Cushing's syndrome, 139
Cushing's syndrome, 139-143
    assessment, 139-141, 140i
    care plan, 142
    intervention, 142-143
    vs. Cushing's disease, 139
Cyproheptadine, 142

D

Demeclocycline, 46
Desiccated thyroid USP, 67
Desmopressin, 42t
Dexamethasone suppression test, 138
Diabetes insipidus, 37, 39-43
    assessment, 39-40
    care plan, 41
    intervention, 41-43
Diabetes mellitus, 95-121
    assessment, 98-100, 102-103
    care plan, 104
    intervention, 103-116
    pathophysiology, 97-98
    signs, 93, 99
    types, 95-97, 96t
Diabetic dermopathy, 102
Diabetic ketoacidosis (DKA), as complication of diabetes mellitus, 116-118, 120t
Diabetic retinopathy, 99, 101i
Diazepam, 128
Diazoxide, 128
Direct testing of hormone levels, 13

E

Edetate disodium (EDTA), role of, in calcium level reduction, 82
Ellsworth-Howard excretion test, 74
Empty-sella syndrome, 30i
Endocrine dysfunction, 10-16
Endocrine glands, 3-16
Endocrine hormones, 3-16
Endocrine principles, 3-16

Enterogastrone, as parahormone, 7
Epinephrine, 132t
Estrogen, 130, 132t
Exercise, as treatment factor in diabetes mellitus, 109, 111
    dietary adjustments for, 110t
    physiologic effects of, 110t
Exocrine glands, 3

F

Fasting blood glucose, 94
Fasting hypoglycemia, 124, 125
    diet therapy for, 128
Feedback mechanism, 7-8, 8i, 9i
    negative
        in parathyroid hormone secretion, 70-71
        in thyroid hormone secretion, 50
Fluid imbalance, assessment of, 46
Follicle-stimulating hormone, 19, 20t
    deficiency, 33
    excess, 32
    levels, measurement of, 28
Follicular carcinoma, 63
Follicular cycle, 24i
Free T_4 index, 56
FSH. *See* Follicle-stimulating hormone.
Furosemide, 46

G

Galactorrhea-amenorrhea syndrome, 32
Gastrin, as parahormone, 7
GH. *See* Growth hormone.
GH stimulation test, 29
GH suppression test, 29
Gigantism, 32
Glipizide, 108, 109
Glucagon, 91, 92t
Glucocorticoids, 130, 132t
Gluconeogenesis, 91
Glucose intolerance disorders, classification of, 96t
Glucose meter, as monitoring technique, 112i
Glucose monitoring, 111-113
Glucose tolerance tests, 94
Glyburide, 108, 109
Glycemic index, 105
Glycogenesis, 91
Glycogenolysis, 91
glycohemoglobin test, 112i, 113
Glycolysis, 91
Glycosylated hemoglobin test, 112i, 113
Goiter, 60
Gonadotropins
    deficiency, 333
    excess, 32
    measurement of, 28
Gonadotropin stimulation test, 28
Graves' disease, 58, 59i
Growth, effects of thyroid hormone on, 51
Growth hormone, 19, 20t
    deficiency, 33
    excess, 32
    levels, measurement of, 28-29
Gull's disease, 64

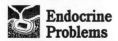

Index

H

Hemoglobin A$_{1c}$ test, 112i, 113
Histamine, as parahormone, 7
Homeostasis
    calcium-phosphate, regulation of, 70
    endocrine system and, 3
Hormones, 3-16
    adrenal, 130, 132t
    classification, 6
    hypothalamic, 19
    pancreatic, 91
    parathyroid, 70-72, 70t
    pituitary, 19-21, 20t
    release and transmission, 6-7
    secretion, 6, 7-8, 8i
    structure and function, 3, 6-10
    thyroid, 48-52, 52t
Hormone-to-hormone regulation, 7-8
Hypercalcemia, 72
    in hyperparathyroidism, 75-77, 79
    intervention, 81-82
Hypercortisolism. *See* Cushing's syndrome.
Hyperglycemia
    signs, 98, 114
Hyperglycemic hyperosmolar nonketotic coma (HHNC), 118-119, 120t, 121
Hypermagnesemia, 83
Hyperparathyroidism, 74-77, 79-82
    assessment, 75-79, 77i
    care plan, 80
    intervention, 79-82
Hyperphosphatemia, 78
Hyperpituitarism, 32
Hyperprolactinemia, 32
Hyperthyroidism, 58-64
    assessment, 58-60, 59i
    care plan, 61
    intervention, 61-63
    vs. hypothyroidism, 53t
Hypocalcemia, 72
    eliciting signs of, 85i
    prevention of, by PTH, 70
Hypoglycemia, 122-129
    assessment, 124-126
    care plan, 127
    as complication of diabetes mellitus, 120t
    hormonal response to, 122t
    intervention, 127-129
    pathophysiology, 123
Hypogonadism, 32
Hypomagnesemia, 83
Hyponatremia, in SIADH, 43, 44i
Hypoparathyroidism, 82-88
    assessment, 84-86
    care plan, 87
    intervention, 87-88
Hypophosphatemia, 78
Hypophysectomy, transsphenoidal, 35, 36i
Hypophysis. *See* Pituitary gland.
Hypopituitarism, 33
Hypothalamic–pituitary–target gland axis, 7-8, 9i
    thyroid hormone regulation and, 50
Hypothalamus, 19
Hypothyroidism, 64-68
    assessment, 64-66, 65i
    care plan, 67
    intervention, 66-67
    vs. hyperthyroidism, 53t

I

Impaired glucose tolerance, 96t
Indirect testing of hormone levels, 13
Indomethacin, 82
Inhibiting factors/hormones, 19
Insulin, 92t
    role of, in blood glucose regulation, 91
    types, 106
Insulin antibody test, 93, 95
Insulin-dependent (Type I) diabetes mellitus, 96-97
    development of, 98
Insulin-induced hypoglycemia, 124
Insulin lipodystrophy, as complication of insulin therapy, 107
Insulinomas, 126
Insulin pumps, 107i
Insulin rebound syndrome, 108
Insulin resistance, 97
Insulin therapy, 105-107
Intermedin, 19, 20t
Interstitial cell–stimulating hormone, 19, 20t
Iodine
    as main component of thyroid hormone, 48
    therapy, 62
Iopanoic acid, 62
Ipodate, 62
Islet cell transplantation, 115i
^{131}I therapy, 62
I.V. glucose tolerance test, 94

K

Ketone bodies, 91
    urine testing for, 111
Ketonemia, as complication of diabetes mellitus, 117
Kocher's test, for tracheal compression, 54

L

Late-stage dumping syndrome, 123-124
LATS. *See* Long-acting thyroid stimulator.
Levothyroxine, 60, 66
LH. *See* Luteinizing hormone.
Liothyronine sodium, 67
Liotrix, 67
Lipogenesis, 91
Lipolysis, 91
Lithium carbonate, 62
Lithium chloride, 46
Long-acting thyroid stimulator, 57
Luteinizing hormone, 19, 20t
    deficiency, 33
    excess, 32
    levels, measurement of, 28
Lypressin, 42t

M

Macroadenomas, 31
Magnesium, 83
    role of, in PTH secretion, 70, 83
Mammotropin, 19, 20t
Mediator mechanism, 6
Medullary carcinoma, 63
Melanocyte-stimulating hormone, 19, 20t
Menstrual hormones, 24i
Metabolism
    calcium/phosphate, role of PTH in, 70
    effects of thyroid hormone on, 51
Methimazole, 51, 61-62
Metyrapone, 142
Metyrapone test, 138
Microadenomas, 31
Mineralocorticoids, 130, 132t, 133
Mitotane, 142
MSH. *See* Melanocyte-stimulating hormone.
Multiple endocrine neoplasia syndrome, 148
Myxedema, 64
Myxedema coma, 66-67

N

Necrobiosis lipoidica diabeticorum, 102
Nelson's syndrome, 142
Nervous system regulation of hormones, 10
Neurohormonal regulation of body fluids, 38i
Neurohypophysis, 4i, 17, 18i
Nodule, solitary thyroid, 60
Non-insulin-dependent (Type II) diabetes mellitus, 97
    development of, 98
Norepinephrine, 132t

O

OGTT. *See* Oral glucose tolerance test.
Oral glucose tolerance test, 94
Organification, iodine, into monoiodotyrosine, 48
Osmolality levels, 38i
Osmoreceptors, function of, 38i
Ovaries, 5i
Ovulation, 24i
Oxidation, iodide, to iodine, 48
Oxytocin, 20-21, 20t

P

Pancreas, 3
    anatomy, 5i, 90i
    endocrine/exocrine function, 90i
Pancreas transplantation, 115i
Pancreatic disorders, 90-129
Pancreatic hormone production, 91
Panhypopituitarism, 31
Paper tape methods of glucose monitoring, 112i

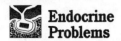
Index

Papillary carcinoma, 63
Paracrine glands, 3
Parahormones, 3, 6, 7
Parathormones, 70-72, 70t
Parathyroid autotransplantation, 81
Parathyroid disorders, 69-88
Parathyroidectomy, 79-81, 81i
Parathyroid glands, anatomy, 4i, 69i
Parathyroid hormones, 70-72, 70t
    calcium regulation and, 72
Pharmacologic hypoglycemia, 124
Phenformin, 109
Pheochromocytoma, 148-153
    assessment, 148-150
    care plan, 150
    intervention, 150-152
Phosphate levels, role of, in PTH regula-
    tion, 70, 78
Phosphates, role of, in calcium level re-
    duction, 82
Pineal gland, 5i
Pituitary apoplexy, 34
Pituitary disorders, 17-46
Pituitary gland
    anatomy, 4i, 17, 18i
    hormone regulation and, 7-8, 9i
Pituitary-hypothalamus relationship, 19
Pituitary infarction, 21
Pituitary insufficiency. See Hypopituita-
    rism.
Pituitary–target gland axis, 7
Pituitary tumors, 30-37
    assessment, 31-34
    care plan, 35
    as cause of visual field loss, 27i
    intervention, 35-37
Plasma C-peptide, 95
Plicamycin, role of, in calcium level re-
    duction, 82
Polydipsia, 40
    psychogenic, 39
Polypeptides, 6
Polyuria, 39-40
Postpartum pituitary gland necrosis,
    26i
Precocious puberty, causes, 11
PRL. See Prolactin.
Prolactin, 19, 20t
    deficiency, 33
    excess, 32
    levels, measurement of, 29
Prolactin secretion test, 29
Propranolol, 61, 62, 128
Propylthiouracil (PTU), 51, 61-62
Prostaglandins, as parahormone, 7
Provocative testing, 13, 15
Pseudohypoparathyroidism, 84
PTH. See Parathyroid hormones.
PTH infusion test, 74

R

Radiation therapy for pituitary tumors,
    36-37
Radioimmunoassay, hormone level mea-
    surement and, 13
Reactive hypoglycemia, 122-124, 125
    diet therapy for, 128
Reagent strip monitoring of glucose lev-
    els, 112i
Releasing factors/hormones, 19

S

Secretin, as parahormone, 7
Serum tests
    for adrenal disorders, 138
    for pancreatic disorders, 95
    for parathyroid disorders, 73
    for pituitary hormone levels, 28-29
    for thyroid disorders, 56-57
Sheehan's syndrome, 26i
SIADH. See Syndrome of inappropriate
    antidiuretic hormone.
Sipple's syndrome, 148
Somatostatin, 92t
Somatotropin, 19, 20t
Somatrem, 35
Somogyi phenomenon, 108
Spironolactone, 142
Steroid(s), 6
    replacement, postoperative, 142
    role of, in calcium level reduction, 82
    therapy, patient teaching for, 146
Stimulation test(s), 13, 15
    ACTH, 183
    thyroid, 56-57
    TRH, 57
Sulfonylurea therapy, 107-109
Sulkowitch's test, 73
Suppression test(s), 13, 15
    dexamethasone, 138
    thyroid, 57
Suprarenal glands. See Adrenal glands.
Syndrome of inappropriate antidiuretic
    hormone, 43-46
    assessment, 45-46
    care plan, 46
    intervention, 46
    pathophysiology, 43, 44i

T

T_3. See Triiodothyronine.
T_4. See Thyroxine.
Testes, anatomy, 5i
Testosterone, 132t
Tetany, in hypoparathyroidism, 84-85
Thymus glands, 5i
Thyroglobulin
    measurement of, 56
    as therapy, 67
Thyroid antibodies test, 57
Thyroid cancer, 63
Thyroid crisis, 61
Thyroid disorders, 48-68
Thyroidectomy, 62-63
Thyroid gland
    anatomy, 4i, 49i
    examination of, 54, 55i
Thyroid hormone, 48-52, 52t
    levels, measurement of, 56-57
Thyroiditis, subacute, 62
Thyroid panel, 55, 57
Thyroid scan (RAIU test), 57
Thyroid-stimulating hormone, 19, 20t
    deficiency, 33
    excess, 32
    levels, measurement of, 28, 56
    role of, in thyroid hormone regulation,
    50

Thyroid storm, 61
Thyroid ultrasound, 58
Thyrotoxicosis, 58-60. See also Hyper-
    thyroidism.
Thyrotropin, 19, 20t
Thyrotropin-releasing hormone (TRH),
    role of, in thyroid hormone regula-
    tion, 50
Thyrotropin-releasing hormone chal-
    lenge, 28, 57
Thyroxine (T_4), 48, 49i, 51, 52t
    levels, measurement of, 56
Thyroxine-binding globulin (TBG), mea-
    surement of, 56
Tolazamide, 108, 109
Tolbutamide, 108, 109
Tolbutamide tolerance, 94-95
Transsphenoidal hypophysectomy, 35,
    36i
Trapping, iodide, 48
T_3 resin uptake, 56
TRH. See Thyrotropin-releasing hor-
    mone.
Triiodothyronine (T_3), 48, 49i, 51, 52t
    levels, measurement of, 56, 57
Trousseau's sign, 85i
TSH. See Thyroid-stimulating hormone.
Tubular reabsorption of phosphate
    (TRP), 73
T_3 uptake ratio, 56
Two-hour postprandial blood glucose, 94

U

Urinary cyclic AMP, 73
Urinary vanillylmandelic acid (VMA),
    138
Urine 17-hydroxycorticosteroids, 138
Urine 17-ketosteroids, 138
Urine metanephrines, 138
Urine specific gravity, 38i
Urine testing
    for glucose monitoring, 111, 112i
    hormone level measurement and, 13

V

Vasopressin, 20-21, 20t
    deficiency, as cause of diabetes insipi-
    dus, 37
    as therapy, 41, 42t
Vasopressin test, 40
Visidex, 112i
Visual field loss, pituitary tumors as
    cause of, 27i
Vitamin D
    as sterol hormone, 74
    therapy, 88

W

Water deprivation test, 29
Water intoxication, SIADH and, 44-45
Wermer's syndrome, 148

i refers to an illustration; t refers to a table